THE AESTHETIC EXPERIENCE OF DYING

Structured around a personal account of the illness and death of the author's partner, Jane, this book explores how something hard to bear became a threshold to a world of insight and discovery.

Drawing on German Idealism and Jane's own research in the area, *The Aesthetic Experience of Dying* looks at the notion of life as a binary synthesis, or a return enhanced, as a way of coming to understand death. Binary synthesis describes the interplay between dynamically opposing pairs of concepts – such as life and death – resulting in an enhanced version of one of them to move forward in a new cycle of the process. Yet what relevance does this elegant word game have to the shocking diagnosis of serious illness? Struggling to balance reason with sense, thought with feeling, this book examines the experience of caring for someone from diagnosis to death and is illustrated with examples of the return enhanced. The concluding chapter outlines how the tension of Jane's dying has been resolved as the rhythmic patterns of the lifeworld have been understood through the process of reflecting on the experience.

This creative and insightful book will appeal to those interested in the medical humanities. It will also be an important reference for practising and student health professionals.

Veronica M. F. Adamson is an Honorary Fellow in the School of Health in Social Science, University of Edinburgh, UK.

'This is a beautiful, visceral and not least courageous text that opens the reader to the depths and details of a human life facing death. Adamson succeeds in offering a poignant reflection that journeys from diagnosis to death in a way that is faithful to the shared depths of the lifeworld. As such, she generously provides a moving and insightful narrative for contemplation about what it is to be human and the nature of the lifeworld in living towards death. It should be read by all professionally involved in terminal illness, it spans insights into well-being, aesthetic dimensions of illness and the implicit splits between reductionist approaches in care delivery and human embodiment which are all skilfully revealed and grasp the human heart.'

Kathleen Galvin, University of Brighton, UK

THE AESTHETIC EXPERIENCE OF DYING

The Dance to Death

Veronica M. F. Adamson

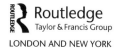

LONDON AND NEW YORK

First published 2018
by Routledge
2 Park Square, Milton Park, Abingdon, Oxon OX14 4RN

and by Routledge
711 Third Avenue, New York, NY 10017

Routledge is an imprint of the Taylor & Francis Group, an informa business

© 2018 Veronica M. F. Adamson

The right of Veronica M. F. Adamson to be identified as author of this work has been asserted by him/her in accordance with sections 77 and 78 of the Copyright, Designs and Patents Act 1988.

All rights reserved. No part of this book may be reprinted or reproduced or utilised in any form or by any electronic, mechanical, or other means, now known or hereafter invented, including photocopying and recording, or in any information storage or retrieval system, without permission in writing from the publishers.

Trademark notice: Product or corporate names may be trademarks or registered trademarks, and are used only for identification and explanation without intent to infringe.

British Library Cataloguing in Publication Data
A catalogue record for this book is available from the British Library

Library of Congress Cataloging in Publication Data
A catalog record for this book has been requested

ISBN: 978-1-138-63522-7 (hbk)
ISBN: 978-1-138-63524-1 (pbk)
ISBN: 978-1-315-20648-6 (ebk)

Typeset in Bembo
by Taylor & Francis Books

For Jane, with love

CONTENTS

Acknowledgements   *viii*
Introduction   *ix*

1   The return enhanced   1
2   Invitation to the dance   43
3   Days for dancing   76
4   The last waltz   116
5   The aesthetic experience of dying   147

Index   *189*

ACKNOWLEDGEMENTS

Writing a book is a solitary task which can lead the author to believe it is solely their unaided achievement. On one level this is true but then there is the network of supporters, encouragers, reviewers and commentators without whom we writers would be a dull and arrogant bunch. So without further ado there are some very important persons, in no particular order, whom I must both acknowledge and thank most sincerely. My wonderful and amazing family – Rose, Sylvain, Wilf and Gélise – are always there to cheer me through the dark, damp bits. Without Margaret, there would have been no Jane and I value greatly her support and friendship. Jane would be so pleased that I continue to dine with her school friends, Anne, Alison and Susan; I am truly grateful for their continuing support and encouragement.

Clodagh Ross provides compassion and friendship while seeking clarity to my obfuscations. My research supervisors, Professor Tonks Fawcett and Dr Marion Smith, guided me when I strayed from the path, as I frequently did, supported my wobbly knees and kept the faith that it could and would be done. The thesis examiners, Dr Rosie Stenhouse and Dr Fiona Cowdell provided apposite comments and suggested reworking the text into a more accessible book format. Rev. Dr Harriet Harris has helped me to explore some of the spiritual aspects of death and dying of the study through a conversation series hosted by the University of Edinburgh Chaplaincy. Grace McInnes at Routledge has provided valuable guidance on the metamorphosis of a thesis into a book. Particular thanks are due to Tonks for her continuing encouragement, draft reviewing and comments especially when she has so many calls on her time.

INTRODUCTION

The realisation that a loved one may be seriously ill is shocking. When those concerns are then confirmed as hard fact, the effect is shattering. From the moment a life-limiting condition is diagnosed, life can and will never be as it had been. Our reactions to such news and its consequences depend on many factors: who it is, what is wrong and our relationship to the person concerned. What we do with this new and unwanted knowledge is dependent on our previous experience, our current circumstances and our worldview of disease and its treatment. Having shared such an experience what then is worthy of formal research? There are possibly two reasons for the justification of studying the experience of caring for someone with life-limiting disease: to make sense of it and to discover if there is anything new to contribute to what is already known. There may also be many other factors in terms of personal interest, unresolved issues and a sense of something unfinished; fundamentally it is the belief that something might need to be better understood.

My partner, Jane, was diagnosed with advanced ovarian cancer in 2011 and died the following May. The time of her illness was one of tension with episodes of intensification as the disease progressed which, for her, was resolved with death. Yet for me there were many questions and uncertainties about what had happened during those months of illness. While I knew her dying had been as she had wished, at home in her own bed, there seemed to be something more to it that I wanted to understand. Or perhaps I was just not yet ready to let her go. Jane had a fine brain, was the first in her family to attend university gaining not just a first but then a PhD. Her doctoral work drew heavily on Goethe and his ideas of secularisation as well as the influence of his relationship with Schiller (Plenderleith, 1991). As a result of her own studies she had formed a view that life could be understood as a *return enhanced* – a way of recognising something that had perhaps been experienced previously but not then fully appreciated. This idea comes from the academic analysis and interpretation of both Schiller's and Goethe's style of writing where concepts are used as dynamically opposing pairs in a style termed *binary synthesis*.

But how could this elegant word game have any relevance or effect on her illness? Through my own doctoral study (Adamson, 2015) I set out to explore what had happened during the time of caring for her from diagnosis to death. As a trained nurse the practicalities were easy; it was dealing with the now very personal nature of the relationship with my *patient* that proved the real challenge. In this book I revisit the doctoral work in a more succinct form and also give some attention to my own journey as a return enhanced to both practical nursing and academia. It will already be apparent that this book is based on a very personal study. As a narrative inquiry of a particular storied world, working with such highly personal stories is fraught with tensions of identity, confidentiality and privacy. While I have no formal evidence from Jane, such as a signed permission document, she did give me her full, unequivocal approval of any research I might do after her death. Our families were also fully aware of the study and their identities are concealed. Having made the decision to retrospectively study our shared experience of Jane's illness and dying, I needed to find an appropriate methodology for the research.

Conventionally phenomenological approaches, particularly Gadamer's hermeneutical phenomenology, would be considered more appropriate to the study of lived experience (van Manen, 1990). But such methods describe a way of being in a particular world for research purposes, of living the experience of such a world. What does the researcher do if they have already had the experience and were not consciously in research mode at the time? Is the answer that the task of phenomenological research and writing is "to construct a possible interpretation of the nature of a certain human experience" (van Manen, 1990: 41)? But I wanted to do more than interpret and explain. While I had no personal need to unravel the detail of specific events and episodes, their sequence is important in order to follow the narrative thread and unfolding story. Nor did I want to reduce the available texts to themes; somehow this work seems to be more than what is written. It was about bearing witness, the testimony of one who walked beside their wounded partner as she resorted to stories of living well to heal the pain of her suffering "As wounded, people may be cared for, but as storytellers, they care for others" (Frank, 2013: xx).

Initially the study was located within my once familiar territory of health care and its principal places of delivery: hospitals and hospices. Now, these familiar places were strange, not just in the sense of the sociological imagination (Wright Mills, 2000) but for me as an actor with a different role from that of the nurse. I had been a nurse who became a carer then researcher and yet these different persona are all part of my being. My conceptualisation of the study was advancing and moving away from what I perceived as the familiar. Now a clinical setting was not just strange but unfamiliar; one where I no longer belonged. As I continued to read and explore possibilities, ideas coalesced around using the materials that I had to hand. This is the potential "bricolage" that can be used in a dialogue with the researcher as "bricoleur" (Levi-Strauss, 1962: 11 & 19). These materials included diaries, notes, email, blog posts and hospital correspondence. The bricolage would be supplemented with my own recollections of the illness period through a series of self-reflective interviews. Inspired by the mixed methods approach suggested in Ken Plummer's *Documents of Life* (2001), I attended a workshop run by Ken himself. I came to realise that by using the existing documents, the research could be centred on the personal experience that had already happened. In addition to the previously identified documents (email correspondence, hospital letters, diaries) and my personal recollections, a third data source was added later when access to the relevant health records was obtained. In the context of narrative medicine "Students of narrative today are committed to close examination not of dead texts but of living textuality and discourse, wherever they may erupt" (Charon, 2006: 41).

A particular issue has been whether the story of Jane's experience, in which I had such a central role, should be conveyed in the third person, as if I was writing about someone else thereby distancing myself. The relationship between author and subject is sharply focused in biographical studies where the position of the researcher is now reflected by the compound term auto/biography to accommodate the relationship "between biography and autobiography, as well as the divisions between self/other, public/private, and immediacy/memory" (Stanley, 1993: 42). Furthermore the role of the researcher and their experience of the research process should be recognised as central and made explicit in the research writing (Stanley & Wise, 1993). These polarities can be considered as binary syntheses, where the ascendency of one can only be seen in the subordination of the other. The significance of the self becomes apparent in respect of others; we can only determine the boundary of private when we give regard to public.

The first few months of any doctoral study are often times of uncertainty, doubt and vacillation as the student struggles with their chosen topic. I certainly wrestled with reconciling my personal experience of death with something more abstract and distanced, and therefore more manageable in terms of academic research. As the idea of personal documents took hold, I made a research note after reading a journal article of Jane's that was based on her thesis (Plenderleith, 1993). For me this was a timely reminder that if Jane's illness was to be the focus of the study, I would also have to address what I understood and perceived to be her core beliefs. That would mean rapidly trying to understand some relatively obscure aspects of eighteenth-century German literature further compounded by ignorance of the language. In a way, it was a kind of hunch that there might be something in Jane's worldview that could account for what I had observed in her apparently graceful death. The result, as the revised version in this book, may at first appear structurally odd but my intention is to first set the scene which includes an introduction to the relationship between two great German dramatists, Goethe and Schiller. They are less well known for their philosophical interests although the collection of Schiller's essays *On the Aesthetic Education of Man* continues to receive some modest attention.

No prior knowledge of the philosophical thinking of Goethe and Schiller and its context in German Idealism is either assumed nor necessary. An explanatory overview is given in the first chapter as part of the background and scene setting. It is here that *The Illness Period*, the eleven months from diagnosis to death, is introduced; the doctoral work began within four months of Jane's death and was completed in three years. The bulk of the book, Chapters 2 to 4, recounts in detail the entire illness experience from when Jane began feeling unwell to her death. The final chapter revisits the three themes: a life limited by illness, aesthetic experience and the return enhanced. The first theme is the central subject which is then considered through the other two. The concept of the return enhanced has also been prominent in the natural cycle of research and writing. The dynamic process of binary synthesis as one of tension, intensity and resolution is set in a wider context. The tension of Jane's dying has been resolved as the rhythmic patterns of the lifeworld have been understood through the process of reflecting on the experience. Yet what had initially seemed a relatively straightforward task of transition from thesis to academic book, has taken longer than anticipated. But as will be seen, it has in itself been a return enhanced.

References

Adamson, Veronica (2015) *The Dance to Death: The Aesthetic Experience of Dying*, PhD Thesis, Edinburgh: University of Edinburgh

Charon, Rita (2006) *Narrative Medicine: Honoring the Stories of Illness*, Oxford: Oxford University Press

Frank, Arthur (2013) *The Wounded Storyteller: Body, Illness, and Ethics*, Chicago: University of Chicago Press, 2nd edition

Levi-Strauss, C (1962) 'The science of the concrete', in C Levi-Strauss, Ed, *The Savage Mind*, Chicago: University of Chicago Press, 1–22

Plenderleith, Helen Jane (1991) *The Testament of Dichtung und Wahrheit: An Enquiry into Goethe's Mode of Secularization*, PhD thesis, Glasgow: University of Glasgow

Plenderleith, Helen Jane (1993) 'An approach to Goethe's treatment of religion in *Dichtung und Wahrheit*', *German Life & Letters*, 46, 297–310

Plummer, Ken (2001) *Documents of Life 2: An Invitation to a Critical Humanism*, London: SAGE

Schiller, Friedrich (2016) *On the Aesthetic Education of Man in a Series of Letters*, Trans. K Tribe, with Notes by A Schmidt, London: Penguin Random House

Stanley, Liz (1993) 'On auto/biography in sociology', *Sociology*, 27, 1, 41–52

Stanley, Liz & Wise, Sue (1993) *Breaking Out Again: Feminist Ontology and Epistemology*, London: Routledge

van Manen, Max (1990) *Researching Lived Experience: Human Science for an Action Sensitive Pedagogy*, Albany: State University of New York Press

Wright Mills, C (2000) *The Sociological Imagination*, Afterword by T Gitlin, Oxford: Oxford University Press

1
THE RETURN ENHANCED

The suggestion that dying and death could be an aesthetic experience may appear crass or insensitive. Yet for those who have time to prepare for their impending demise, it can be a rich and rewarding experience. A terminal diagnosis is overwhelming in its first visceral impact but then eases into a background portent of inevitability. The chapter is in three sections. In the first part, "Invitation to the dance", I outline how Jane and I came to be together and share a path through life and work. Our common interest in polarity or binary synthesis was based for Jane on the philosophical thinking of the German polymaths, Goethe and Schiller. To understand the essence of Jane, there is a detailed explanation in part two of binary synthesis and the return enhanced through the "Influence of German Idealism". These have become pivotal to my understanding and interpretation of the illness experience. The final part, "Research aesthetics", provides an overview of the methods used to gather and formalise the study data.

Part one: invitation to the dance

Jane was diagnosed in the July; the treatment plan was chemotherapy then surgery. The reality was some respite then rapid decline and she died the following May. As those few statements suggest the story is primarily about her illness and death but they were also a catalyst to investigate some of the more abstract layers which emerged from the basic facts. It is not uncommon for the bereaved to throw themselves into some new, time consuming enterprise. To use the experience as a basis for academic research is perhaps more unusual but not necessarily invalid. While training as a nurse and during my subsequent nursing practice I had cared for many women with gynaecological cancers; these were my companion stories (Frank, 2010). Such accounts accompany us through life, acting as a guidance system assisting with our reactions to events or circumstances. However, my gynaecological companion stories were not helpful friends; they were harbingers of doom acting as constant reminders of the destructive and disfiguring nature of such cancers. Or at least they did not at first appear to be friends until I came to realise that although they foretold of difficult, unpleasant endings, that very knowledge was empowering. I was forewarned and could therefore be forearmed when that time surely came for Jane.

At various times during the course of the research, others assumed that the study might be autoethnographic, a term used in reference to "autobiographies that self-consciously explore the interplay of the introspective, personally engaged self with cultural descriptions mediated through language, history, and ethnographic explanation" (Ellis & Bochner 2000: 742). Suggestions were made of studies such as personal bereavement following a father's unexpected death (Sehn, 2013) or the earlier traumatic loss of a brother (Ellis, 1993). But the study was not about sudden or unanticipated bereavement; I knew the ending from the outset, and did not want the research to be autoethnographic. While I accepted my role and position as a personally engaged self was central, I was not the principal character or focus of attention; that privilege was for Jane. However, I did and do recognise my role as the researcher and reflexive agent in the unfolding narrative. The methodology that emerged from the original study is detailed elsewhere (Adamson, 2015) while the account given here is limited to an explanation of the basic process and the principal data sources – the stories.

The doctoral research attempted to understand the stories that were told as a direct result of the illness experience. Essentially there were three categories of story: those written by Jane herself; those told about Jane; and my own recollections of events. Jane's stories were the 'official' version of her illness and its progression as told through our personal blog. The 'real version' of these stories about Jane were exchanged between clinicians in their various roles. We had verbal accounts from hospital visits and when we did have something written they were copies of letters addressed to our general practitioner (GP). But the third category of the central story was the one that filled me to overflowing and drove me to research the sorry episode. The drive to narrate experience is, as Rita Charon has observed "to tell and simultaneously listen to a story that reflects and constitutes the self" (Charon, 2006: 74). Ultimately the study was the final act of caring, one last thing I could do to honour my partner and our suffering, to learn from our shared experience. Going deeper and deeper into a painful story is not easy or comfortable but ultimately it is justified as the tension of the research is resolved through understanding and finding peace.

An earlier dance

I qualified as a general nurse in 1979 and worked in various positions as a staff nurse before becoming the ward sister of a general medical ward. An interest in education and research led to a nursing research training fellowship with the intention of studying the conceptualisation of nursing as a profession in its transition from ephemeral art to quantifiable science. Being registered for a PhD without a first degree proved to be beyond my capabilities at the time; I withdrew from academia and also from nursing. After retraining as a software engineer, a career in further and higher education progressed from lecturer to independent consultant. It was during the latter part of this time that I first met Jane in a professional context. All that we experienced was perceived as an opportunity for learning and mutual enrichment. Together, we had arrived at an interplay between thinking and doing, theory and practice by very different routes: Jane through her own doctoral study of secularisation in Goethe's autobiographical writing (Plenderleith, 1991) and mine through adult education and systems analysis (Adamson, 1999).

We met when we were both employed in a major higher education initiative to establish a university for the Scottish Highlands and Islands. When the project became a reality we moved on and created our own educational consultancy specialising in the use of learning technologies to support tertiary education. It operated with modest success for more than ten years, advising colleges and universities across the United Kingdom (UK). After some intense years of working predominantly through government agencies, we were becoming tired and jaded. Political changes were likely with a shift of the UK's administrative powers from centre left to centre right; there was also the banking crisis and its consequent austerity measures. By the autumn of the year preceding Jane's diagnosis, we had decided to sell our house, put necessities in store and pack essentials (including two cats) into an estate car and a small caravan. We headed for Eastern France in a bitterly cold winter. Our intention, once we were settled, was partly to start a small gardening enterprise but mostly to enjoy a European life in France, bordering Germany with a view of Switzerland. We felt sure our enthusiasm and Jane's fluency in both French and German were sufficient to ensure success.

The following March we were back in Scotland, older, wiser and ready for the next challenge: where to live. Then, just as we thought we could start to enjoy life in Edinburgh, Jane was rather surprisingly diagnosed with ovarian cancer. It was surprising because we both believed ourselves to be fit and healthy, with a lifestyle grounded by a good diet and plenty of exercise. With hindsight, it did perhaps explain her lack of energy and dwindling enthusiasm abroad. It was not simply weariness of consultancy work, she was seriously ill yet apparently innocent of her condition. Our way of being, when faced with this most difficult of life challenges was not to dwell on why Jane had cancer, nor when she might die from the disease but to live what remaining life we had together in a state of Voltairean optimism "everything was for the best, in the best of all possible worlds" (Voltaire, 2008: 4). The influence of *Candide* continued with the shared attitude that this great tragedy would be faced with humour. This is well illustrated by one of Jane's last diary entries, when eating and drinking had become severely compromised and the morphine parched her mouth 'Wouldn't you just die for lemon sorbet?'.

Pas de deux

Our mutual attraction was confirmed with the realisation that we had arrived, by very different routes, at a shared understanding: a whole is more than the sum of its parts. For Jane this is best exemplified in her doctoral thesis (Plenderleith, 1991) where she explores secularisation in Goethe's *Dichtung und Wahrheit* (Poetry and Truth). I have little understanding of German and therefore had only a general appreciation of her study. However, I knew from years of living and working with her that the methodological tool she had used in her research was central to her understanding and conceptualisation of her world. This certainty and epistemological confidence may seem too strong but I will demonstrate the evidence is there in both her writing and attitude to her own mortality. The conventional approach to biography is through microscopic examination of all available materials. In realising that biographical work is equally autobiographical, it is actually kaleidoscopic "each time you look, you see something different, composed certainly of the same elements, but in a new configuration" (Stanley, 1992: 158). Accordingly, I draw here on both the material evidence I have that could be examined by any researcher and my personal, and therefore unique, knowledge of Jane and her life. My memories are the jewel patterns of a kaleidoscope and not the penetrating spotlight of a microscope.

Goethe's autobiography is a refashioning of his recollections (*Dichtung*) and factual information (*Wahrheit*) (Mahoney, 2002). The essence of Jane's argument was that "Goethe's treatment of religion in *Dichtung und Wahrheit* may best be approached as a representation of sacral principles in secular form, as an interaction of these polarised opposites, by the methodological tool of binary synthesis" (Plenderleith, 1993: 297). It is this quotation that introduces in a single, albeit complex, sentence Jane's worldview. I will not pretend that I fully understand, despite her best efforts to explain, the nuanced meaning she drew from her study of Goethe's discussion of religion. What I do know is that it led her to part company with her Christian upbringing, to accept her own sexuality, and for her conceptual understanding of life to be in terms of a virtuous interplay between opposing poles. Binary synthesis is essentially the interaction of two different concepts from which a third concept can emerge. This third concept is distinct in itself but contains all the elements of the other two within it. What appealed to Jane is the realisation that there is an inherent relationship between any pair of oppositional concepts. As a simple example, a question can exist but it needs an answer. Once a question has an answer it becomes subordinated to it in a process where they can then both be subordinated to or enhanced by the other.

Jane made extensive use of this mode of analysis, identified by the translators of Schiller's *On the Aesthetic Education of Man*[1] (Wilkinson & Willoughby, 1967)[2], in her own thesis (Plenderleith, 1991). It is on this basis and my personal knowledge of Jane's regular reference to *binary synthesis* or her own preferred term, 'a return enhanced', that I believe this mode of thought to be central to her personal philosophy. The essence is exemplified in Goethe's famous maxim that "There is nothing worth thinking but it has been thought before; we must only try to think again" (Goethe, 1906: 1). An earlier thought or understanding is enhanced by new information and insights. A more precise explanation of binary synthesis and its origins follows later in this chapter.

In the dissertation for my Master's degree in adult education (Adamson, 1999), I chose to investigate what was perceived then as a paradigm shift in post-compulsory education. The shift was towards student-centred learning, which had started with John Dewey and the notion of lifelong learning and the subsequent move towards experiential learning (Jarvis, 1995: 17). At that time I became aware of the work of Fritjof Capra and his exploration of the parallels between modern physics and eastern mysticism. The statement of the Taoist principle "that any pair of opposites constitutes a polar relationship where each of the two poles is dynamically linked to the other" (Capra, 1975: 114) led to a shift in my thinking. The polarity inherent within the educational paradigm that results from apparently opposing views should not be perceived as a problem but as a potential for change. It was only when Jane read my dissertation that she realised the similarity between our two philosophical approaches to life. We were both driven to see polarities not in a dualistic sense but through their holistic relationship. We were not consciously choosing to adopt a particular philosophical orientation to our lives together but it was part of our mutual attraction. Nehamas, in his consideration of *The Art of Living*, is not recommending a return to classical Greece but the recognition of a philosophical basis to a particular worldview, "The sort of self one constructs as a result of adopting certain theories is not simply a biographical matter. It is, much more importantly, a literary and philosophical accomplishment" (Nehamas, 1998: 2). If we take the time to understand a perspective for ourselves and not simply follow the way of our upbringing, then some intellectual accomplishment may also be derived from the effort. Our unity was brokered through binary synthesis, it was our common thread.

Dancing metaphors

The choice of the word 'dance' in the title is with figurative intent. I use the meaning and organisation of dance in a general sense to illustrate what I perceived as the disruption created by illness to an otherwise orderly, shared life. It had emerged quite naturally during *The Illness Period*. One particular day I became very aware of how our life together had become a series of dances, little step sequences, between the GP's surgery, the chemotherapy day unit and the hospital clinic; we danced attendance to the health professionals' tune. At times it was complicated and required the best of my logistical skills and forward planning, primarily to protect Jane from such necessary trivia. Yet it was also a time of joy, of small triumphs and simple enjoyment. To wallow in the impending gloom of her approaching death seemed a wilful waste of such precious time.

Initially I interpreted this as a loss of control and self-determination (Nordgren & Fridlund, 2001) and later as the temporal, medical disruption to our autonomy (Frankenberg, 1988). Then I remembered an image my sister, who is a printmaker, had sent me during the illness, of a naked, dancing woman that appears on the book cover. That realisation and subsequent visualisation of a female form moving through light and dark, became an iconic metaphor for the study and its particular conceptualisation of the illness experience. The use of metaphor in everyday life and language are commonplace "Metaphorical concepts provide ways of understanding one kind of experience in terms of another kind of experience" (Lakoff & Johnson, 1980: 486). In this sense the metaphor is clearly a useful figurative device to write or talk about difficult or sensitive topics such as death, dying and disease. Consequently, the use of metaphor in relation to illness and especially cancer, is frequent both in terms of the disease process itself and in the course of the illness (Fawcett, 2011).

Susan Sontag was taken to the "kingdom of the ill" (Sontag, 1978: 3) by her cancer and wrote polemically about her experience not just of her illness but of the stigmatisation of disease. In doing so she framed our understanding of metaphors for disease and the experience of illness in the twentieth century (Clow, 2001). For some, Sontag's stand against the use of metaphor has been welcomed as they came to terms with their own disease. Sontag's (1978) *Illness as Metaphor*, has been described as "an eloquent plea against metaphorical thinking in matters medical" (Stacey, 1997: 45) but also recognises that it is the power of metaphor that "makes the silence speak" (Stacey, 1997: 64). A contrasting view of Sontag that recognises the biological symptoms of illness, also sees the "coded metaphors that speak to the contradictory aspects of social life, expressing feelings, sentiments, and ideas that must be otherwise kept hidden" (Scheper-Hughes & Lock, 1986: 138). Using metaphors to tell the story of the disease and its processes provides a means for the ill person to distance themselves from the reality of their situation. The focus of the metaphor is on the disease, the illness and the effect upon the person and their illness experience (Pierret, 2003). Metaphors are also coping strategies for the emotional work of nurses in caring for the dying through both bodily containment and distancing such as "switching on and off" (Froggatt, 1998: 335).

The dance of death appears in many European cultures, most often as the *dance macabre* (French) but also as *Totentanz* (German), as an allegory for the universality of death, usually as a grotesque image but also in writing and music. Its origin has been traced to a now lost mural in the Parisian *Cimetière des Innocents* which depicted the fatal encounter of the living with death personified. It is a memento mori, literally remember you must die. Through a variety of metaphors and formats the meaning remains clear: death comes to us all regardless of age, gender or rank (Oosterwijk & Knöll, 2011). Such representations are deliberately dark and intentionally morbid, nothing to do with the light frivolity of dance. Janesick (1998) employs the metaphor of dance to describe her process of qualitative research, identifying three distinct stages: warm-up, exercises and cool-down. In this study the dance metaphor is expanded to give a choreographic insight into the relationship and interplay between the carer as choreographer and the cared for, who is both dancer and director of the dance as it progresses. The metaphor also serves as a reminder of binary synthesis as the interplay of opposites.

My purpose in using the metaphor of dance is also an attempt to surface a lighter, more playful touch towards illness, disease and suffering which reflects our shared experience. There were some desperate, dark moments, but there was far more light, play and fun. Writing as a method of inquiry has been practised since the seventeenth century by both those concerned with science and the arts, despite the respective associations with objective truth and subjective falsehood (Richardson, 2000). Within the social sciences the use of metaphor is everywhere "Metaphors organise social scientific work and affect the interpretations of the 'facts'; indeed, facts are interpretable ('make sense') only in terms of their place within a metaphoric structure" (Richardson, 2000: 927). But metaphors are not the only trope, those words and phrases which are used in figurative language to create an image (as a visualisation) of something over and above its actual meaning. Metaphor, where reality is framed through analogy when a figure of speech enables us to see one thing in terms of another, is the most widely used trope (Chandler, 2002: 124). In addition to metaphor, other tropes are used in the figurative language of illness writings:

> notwithstanding Sontag's passionate argument against metaphor, many medical anthropologists would contend that it is impossible to think of illness except by means of tropes. Progress occurs by merely replacing one metaphor with a less inadequate one.
>
> *(Lambek, 2003: 6)*

Perhaps more importantly in this context, irony has a special place with regard to illness and treatment where irony may be foregrounded by the illness situation, or at least its recognition, and that therapeutic discourse may be understood by the extent to which irony is recognised. "Irony is thus both an element of self-knowledge and a perspective on it. Illness and treatment sometimes either ignore or objectify and exaggerate the will and agency of sufferers" (Lambek, 2003: 16). For example, when Jane became bald during chemotherapy she quipped that she was 'too sexy for my hair'.[3] This point is also recognised in teaching medical students where irony may be relevant in the narrative writing of clinical settings. It gives distance to the author enabling them to use it when "nearing a truth that is too painful to say" (Charon, 2006: 170). It affords us the bittersweet option, a way to tell the nasty nice.

Part two: the influence of German Idealism

During the original study I realised the work might not just be a personal resolution to Jane's untimely end, or a validation of my nursing efforts but it might also address what we had intended to do once we had time, probably in retirement. It had been our plan to work on a publication that brought together holistic inquiry with the spirit of German Idealism, a term which is fraught with attempts at a precise definition yet what "all its forms have in common is the attempt to save criticism from skepticism, and naturalism from materialism" (Beiser, 2005: 18). All the difficult German stuff would be explained to me by Jane and together we would bring some of the idealised spirit of the eighteenth century to my understanding of systems. If I am honest, we would probably have never found the time, inclination or tenacity to complete such a task, being too busy with daily life. An additional justification that connects with the interests of a wider audience is suggested by this quotation from a book published after the study began:

> The transformational experiences of dying people commonly reorient their attention toward their own inner life. A fresh and growing appreciation of the outer life around them emerges as a result. This reorientation to the inner life is a counterbalance to their usual sense of living with a contracting sense of time and gives them a sense of growing depth.
>
> *(Kellehear, 2014: 214)*

So in order to have some appreciation and understanding of Jane's personal philosophy as the narrative unfolds, some knowledge of her intellectual experience would be helpful. It would of course have been much easier if, as a linguist, she had followed a more conventional path such as being a school teacher. Then it would have been easy to include a few choice quotations from Voltaire, Flaubert, Schiller and Goethe. But no, she spent seven years studying Goethe and Schiller, not just in Scotland, but also in Germany at their University of Jena, and in Weimar, home to Goethe. So, as the late sociologist Ian Craib entreated:

> When we talk about a person who is dying we need to know at least something about their history and character (otherwise, ... we might end up attributing that person's normal attitudes to the fact that they are dying) and we need to know something about the experience of dying (292). ... There is a psychological and a philosophical dimension to our understanding of death and I think these are more important than the sociological, if only because they enable a critique of contemporary social scripts and roles that surround dying.
>
> *(Craib, 2003: 295)*

In this second part of the chapter there is first a brief contextualisation of eighteenth-century Germany and a brief overview of the philosophy of Immanuel Kant. The relationship between Schiller and Goethe is introduced followed by an account of Schiller's ideas of aesthetic education. The common understanding between the two men is illustrated through an outline of Goethe's scientific studies and his conception of the Urphenomenon or primal phenomenon. Finally, there is an interpretation of binary synthesis and the return enhanced. There is no attempt to replicate or examine Jane's own scholarly contribution to Goethe's treatment of religion in his autobiographical works (Plenderleith, 1991).

Germany in the eighteenth century

Any philosophical movement needs to be understood in its historical context (Beiser, 2005) and this is certainly true of German Idealism. In the eighteenth century, towards the end of the Enlightenment or Age of Reason, advances in knowledge were no longer based on Christian faith but on scientific understanding. In Europe this was not simply due to scientific advancement but a societal change following the Thirty Years War and the 1648 Treaty of Westphalia (Croxton, 1999). The treaty included the first recorded use of the word 'secularisation' to indicate the transfer of both power and land from the church to the state (Plenderleith, 1993). War and societal upheaval continued in Europe from 1792 with the French Revolution and continued through the Napoleonic wars which finally ended in 1815.

Despite the disruption and decimation of war, inspired by the environment of philosophical idealism, German Romanticism emerged as a significant literary movement. German scholars are more specific and refer to this as German or Weimar Classicism embodied by the works of Johann Wolfgang Goethe (1749–1832) and Friedrich Schiller (1759–1805) (Brown, 2009). Jane provides a succinct definition of Weimar Classicism as a general programme in "re-presenting known truths, inherited knowledge and wisdom, in a new, dynamised and revitalised form which invites their re-appraisal" (Plenderleith, 1993: 309). In recent years the relevance and significance of the contribution made by both German Idealism and Romanticism have been recognised not least because they can now be seen as grounded in the more modern idea of human freedom (Redding, 2011). Another feature of the movement was its interdisciplinary nature that transcended traditional academic boundaries. Its works continue to influence other fields such as the humanities in general and more specifically art, literary theory and religious studies (Ameriks, 2000). The 250th anniversary of Goethe's birth in 1999 (Sharpe, 2002) and the bicentennial anniversary of Schiller's death in 2005 (Craig, 2005) produced a plethora of publications and renewed interest not just in their works but in the wider movement.

By the latter half of the eighteenth century the German philosopher Immanuel Kant (1724–1804) in his attempt to bridge the gap between rationalism and empiricism (Richards, 2002), had published three critiques on reason and judgement where he developed his system of transcendental realism. Essentially he determined that we can only know the world through our experience of phenomena (as sensed). This perception through ideas and not through material substance, is known as idealism (Redding, 2011). Aesthetics is now generally understood to be the philosophical appreciation of beauty and art but despite the section title of *Transcendental Aesthetics* in the *Critique of Pure Reason* (1781), Kant is really referring to his conceptualisation of sensual experience. It is only in his later work, *The Critique of Judgement* (1790), that his inquiry shifts to the consideration of taste in terms of beauty and art (Hammermeister, 2002).

The relevance of Kant and his understanding of form, matter and aesthetics here is that his work informed and stimulated other writers and philosophers in both Germany and Britain at that time. In an attempt to unify the distinctly theoretical and practical parts of Kant's philosophy, Fichte[4] had devised a system of idealist philosophy, *Wissenschaftslehre*, or a doctrine of science. He wanted to show that from a single, unifying principle came sensibility and understanding as the form and content of experience. Fichte gave Schiller an advance copy of his essay with its theme of reciprocal causality (Dahlstrom, 2000). As will be seen, this idea was later to become a central theme for Schiller's philosophical writings. Despite initial success, the subjective idealism of both Kant and Fichte gave way to the increasing criticism of the younger romantic philosophers, particularly Schelling and Hegel, who proposed a doctrine of absolute idealism, *Naturphilosophie*, or a philosophy of nature (Beiser, 2005). However, although Schiller was aware of these ideas, his interest remained with Kant's attempt to find transcendental principles for aesthetics. Yet these were simply reflections of a knowing subject on given forms; the dependency of the imagination on spatial and temporal constructs. Schiller wanted a more holistic appreciation that could account for the contemplation of beauty as a transitory path from nature to morality (Dahlstrom, 2000).

Goethe and Schiller

In the midst of this philosophical flux Schiller arrived as a young military physician and successful playwright, to take up a post at the University of Jena (Reed, 2002). Schiller was born into a military family and despite his desire to become a pastor, when he was 13 his father enrolled him as a cadet at the military academy or Karlsschule, founded by his patron Karl Eugen, Duke of Württemberg. It was the Karlsschule who assigned him to a medical training as one more suited to his temperament and to provide greater intellectual satisfaction. A particular strength of the curriculum was philosophy and the debates in aesthetics, moral philosophy and literature were to have a lasting impression (Sharpe, 1991). On completion of his studies in 1780, Schiller was discharged from the academy but not from military service. He had already had his first play, *The Robbers*, written while on sickbay night duty, performed with modest success which left no desire to be a poorly salaried regimental physician (Sharpe, 1991; Craig, 2005). In 1782 he deserted and escaped to stay with friends who supported him through his itinerant years until he found fame. By chance, at a performance of his *Don Carlos* in Weimar, he met Goethe's patron, Karl August, who appointed him councillor (Craig, 2005).

Schiller had greatly admired Goethe in his youth but an early meeting while he was a cadet had not been propitious; Schiller found his idol to be egoistic and unapproachable. He was also envious of Goethe's easy rise to fame through his fortuitous personal and social circumstances. While Schiller recognised Goethe's poetic genius, the older man was unimpressed by the younger's wildness and deep commitment to Kant's abstraction (Reed, 2002). Despite these misgivings, Goethe found Schiller a position as professor of history at the University of Jena. Following his two year absence from Weimar while he toured Italy, Goethe returned and found himself disconnected from the Weimar circle. He needed someone highly intelligent to talk to and Schiller wanted a supporter for his new literary journal, *Die Horen* (The Graces). In 1794, a formal invitation to join the journal led to their first real meeting, an awkward encounter which confirmed their differences "Goethe's commitment to empirical realities as against Schiller's to mental structures" (Reed, 2002: 102). However, despite their apparent differences Schiller persevered and sent an emollient letter[5] emphasising their common ground in cultural history and literature. He proposed that their divergent views were in fact complementary and therefore of mutual benefit. Fortuitously the letter arrived in time for Goethe's birthday; their ensuing deep friendship lasted until Goethe was shattered by Schiller's premature death in 1805 causing him to write "I am losing half of my existence" (Reed, 2002: 103). In the birthday letter Schiller sets out the typological differences between them, suggesting that Goethe's approach is one of synthesis whereas his own is more theoretical. A letter the following week further elaborates his theory:

> Your mind works intuitively to an extraordinary degree, and all your thinking powers appear, as it were, to have come to an agreement with your imagination to be their common representative ... My understanding works more in a symbolising method, and thus I hover, as a hybrid, between ideas and perceptions, between law and feeling, between a technical mind and genius.
> (Schmitz, 1877: 12)

These and many other letters (Schmitz, 1877, 1890) between the two men are testament to their genuine friendship and the reciprocal nature of their respective characters. Three years later Goethe acknowledges the significance of their relationship in a letter to Schiller, "You have taught me to look at the many-sidedness of the inner man more fairly, you have given me a second youth and re-fashioned me into a poet, which I may be said to have ceased to be" (Schmitz, 1890: 6). During the decade of their friendship the production of both men was prolific: Goethe made great progress with both his longstanding projects, *Faust* and *Wilhelm Meister*, while Schiller wrote many plays including *Maria Stuart* and *Wilhelm Tell*. And Goethe's influence in Schiller's great philosophical project on the aesthetics of humanity has also been acknowledged (Wilkinson & Willoughby, 1967). An elegant interpretation of their relationship with particular relevance in this context is suggested by Reed (2002: 112):

> If the formula 'living form' in Schiller's account of beauty sums up the aesthetic ideal of the Goethe–Schiller collaboration, their attempt to integrate opposites, then the ethical core of their partnership is the idea of overcoming those 'subjective limits' and learning to live with difference.

To understand beauty as life itself in all its rough rawness, is to appreciate life with all its polarities and imperfections.

Schiller and aesthetics

Troubled by the French Revolution, Schiller recognised that his interest in aesthetics might seem to be at odds with the turmoil of the political world. However, he argued that his focus on aesthetics was *for* the sake of politics as freedom could be found on the path to beauty (Beiser, 2005). Schiller's enthusiasm had been sparked by his desire to find objectivity in Kant's *Critique of Judgement*. While he concurred with Kant's distinction of the beautiful from things or objects, defining aesthetics as a judgement of beauty necessitated some challenges (Wilkinson & Willoughby, 1967). He spent two years exploring the nature of beauty, then the moral and the aesthetic as the beautiful soul and finally the nature of the individual in society (Schaper, 1985). Schiller's insights and ideas on each of these themes were published as a series of letters and as an essay, the principal way at the time to inform aesthetic discourse. The development of philosophical aesthetics in Germany, at this time when it was not a unified country but a series of individual states and principalities, resulted from two key factors (Hammermeister, 2002). First, there was resistance to communication with and in other languages; therefore philosophical discussions maintained an internal purity. Second, although German developments were self-sufficient, others responded without actually influencing them. The direct influence of the German aesthetic tradition can be traced down through German philosophers, for example, the emergence of phenomenology from Husserl, Heidegger and Gadamer. It is also an influence on the work of others such as Merleau-Ponty, Sartre and Ricoeur (Hammermeister, 2002).

In 1792 Schiller wrote to his close friend Christian Gottfried Korner, with whom he had lodged for a time in Leipzig, of his epiphany after studying Kant's *Critique of Pure Judgement*. He wanted to clarify his insights into the nature of beauty as an objective of taste, as previously doubted by Kant (Beiser, 2005). Schiller intended to overcome the Kantian dualism of nature and freedom, and the latter's insistence that morality lay in obedience which seemed to Schiller to be "a lamentable gulf between feeling and action, a denial of the possibility of the harmonious personality" (Sharpe, 1991: 135). His ideas would be explicated through his plan to write a book, in dialogue form, that he would call *Kallias*[6] (Schindler, 2008). Illness and other commitments intervened and the book was never written. However, in early 1793 Schiller did maintain a dialogue as a series of letters with Korner which were posthumously published in 1847 as the *Kalliasbriefe* (*Kallias Letters*) (Bernstein, 2002; Schindler, 2008). Recalling the earlier point regarding the introspective nature of German aestheticism, the development of a philosophical argument through correspondence may seem at odds with any genuine scholarly purpose. The epistolary letter form was popular at the time (Schaper, 1985) and it has now been recognised as having scholarly value (Stanley, 2012), but it may well have served to undermine and undervalue Schiller's efforts. Despite the considerable contribution made by Schiller to modern understandings of aesthetics, he is best remembered as a poet and playwright (Beiser, 2005; Craig, 2005) and not as a philosopher.

Schiller believed that aesthetics were important to daily life both publicly and privately, particularly with regard to community living. However, despite his educative intentions, he provides little discussion of art and while making much of beauty, his interest is more with the notion of the beautiful (Schaper, 1985). His purpose was to propose an alternative to both enlightenment and revolution which he argued had failed to overcome the ills of society. His solution was to encourage a movement towards the notion of the ideal as "a unifying moment of reason and feeling, beauty and morality" (Hammermeister, 2002: 49). The way for humanity to achieve this ideal was through the enhancement of everyday life which would not only be easier, it would become "the good life" (Schaper, 1985: 156). At the heart of Schiller's argument is a return enhanced to what he perceived as the natural state of classical Greek culture intensified through a renewed appreciation of modern life. The tension from Schiller's earlier attempts to reconcile beauty and morality are finally resolved in his *Aesthetic Letters*.[7] The central concept of the treatise is that the play-impulse is the basis for all art and is the foundation for "the much more difficult art of living".[8] The solution lies in understanding aesthetic education as the mediator between sense and intellect (Schaper, 1985); a holistic process of personal self-development while being active in community life.

During a period of ill health in 1791 and to free him of his responsibilities as an unsalaried professor, Schiller was awarded a stipend by Prince Friedrich Christian, Duke of Augustenburg. The pension gave him the freedom to pursue his philosophical studies. By 1793 he sent his preliminary thoughts as a sort of progress report to his patron hence the first letter begins "I have, then, your gracious permission to submit the results of my inquiry concerning Art and Beauty in the form of a series of letters."[9] The complete set of twenty seven letters were first published in 1795 as three separate parts in his journal *Die Horen* (Wilkinson & Willoughby, 1967). Despite Goethe's approval, the response to the *Aesthetic Letters* was at best ambivalent (Schaper, 1985). The reaction is unsurprising; the text is metaphysical and difficult to understand. Some (Kimball, 2001) have suggested Snell's (Schiller, 1954) earlier translation more suited to the general reader than Wilkinson and Willoughby's (1967) scholarly edition with its dense text, mixed page numbering, and parallel translation augmented by a commentary, glossary and various appendices. Despite all the 'help', "The letters are a difficult work to digest, and even the most sympathetic reader is often left baffled" (Schaper, 1985: 160). But I was innocent then of such opinions. All I knew was Jane's well-thumbed copy of the Wilkinson and Willoughby translation[10] with its countless pencil annotations and bought in 1983 when she started her doctoral studies. It seemed to be permeated with her spirit and so I persevered with the complexity. My first attempts and understanding (Adamson, 2015) now seem a muddle of emerging ideas, concepts and a grasping sense of bewilderment. What I am trying to do now is present a clearer and more explanatory account of the *Aesthetic Letters* as their relevance and apposite content have become more apparent. Crucially this concerns both the form and the content of the text.

Schiller's aim in the *Aesthetic Letters* is to present in an elegant fashion the two aspects of the psyche,[11] sense and reason, in a process of mutual subordination and interplay from which a third 'play' drive emerges. Schiller's approach can be summarised as a simple formula which begins by

> first analysing human beings down to their basic elements, the opposed impulses to form and to matter, which art can reconcile in free play. The

integration of abstract and concrete, reflection and embodiment, which Schiller demands of art thus corresponds to the most fundamental human need and could restore lost psychic, social and ultimately even political balance.

(Reed, 2002: 109)

However, as the entire text is structured in oppositional pairs which are mediated by a third term (Hammermeister, 2002), the simple formula is not immediately apparent. Nor is it clear if "'aesthetic education' meant for Schiller 'education through' or 'education to' the aesthetic" (Schaper, 1985: 153). Wilkinson and Willoughby insist (and Jane has underlined) that it is both "education *from* the aesthetic through the aesthetic to the aesthetic".[12] His goal is a demonstration of moral harmony both in the form or management of his writing and the actual content or material. The extensive study of the *Aesthetic Letters* undertaken by Wilkinson and Willoughby (1967), reveal them to be a complex work with mathematical proportions, where regular intervals of three are used to develop the central tenet of a 'third thing'.[13] Schiller develops his argument and theory of drives (Hammermeister, 2002) through the twenty seven letters, a number which may seem odd or even arbitrary. However, the aesthetic was not just confined to the content of the letters but also in the presentation of the text. There is a geometric, rhythmic pattern in the articulation of his ideas in both the relationship between the letters and in the actual phrasing of the text as binary syntheses. While many have presented an analysis and overview of the *Aesthetic Letters* (Grossman, 1968; Schaper, 1985; Sharpe, 1991; Dahlstrom, 2000; Hammermeister, 2002; Beiser, 2005) it is only Wilkinson and Willoughby who outlined the symmetrical three–nine relationship between the letters. Their purpose is not to found speculation on the 'significance of number-symbolism'[14] but to highlight the circular and not linear movement in the structure of Schiller's argument, a deliberate ploy to keep the reader's mind moving.

In addition to the structural framework of the letters, Schiller also played various language games in the actual text such as using tautology as with the third thing, and chiasmus between antithetical word pairs. A simple example of a chiasmus is in John F Kennedy's inaugural address when he said "ask not what your country can do for you; ask what you can do for your country" (Kennedy, 1961). The terms 'your country' and 'you' in the first phrase are inverted or switched in the second. What Schiller does is more complex using two contrasting ideas such as matter and form or feeling and reason, switching them to represent the tension that can arise in the interplay between two such concepts. The constructs are used to describe the mediating behaviours or drives, of aesthetic man between ideal and natural man. Schiller drew on Fichte's theory of reciprocity to elaborate freedom as coordinate between and not subordinate of, one drive with the other (Dahlstrom, 2011). The drives can be understood as man's powers, faculties or forces (Wilkinson & Willoughby, 2002).

The essence of Schiller's argument appears in *Letter 12*[15] where he identifies two basic drives: first the *Stofftrieb* or *sense-drive*, concerned with material reality and sensation; secondly, the *Formtrieb* or *form-drive* is concerned with rational necessity and morality. The tension between these polarities calls for a third drive, first appearing in *Letter 15*[16] as the *Spieltrieb* or *play-drive*. In *Letter 18*, beauty becomes the objective of this third drive:

> Beauty links the two opposite conditions of feeling and thinking; yet between these two there is absolutely no middle term. The former truth we know from Experience; the latter is given to us directly by Reason.[17]

A contemporary, albeit somewhat simplified, interpretation of the two drives is that the sense-drive can be perceived as a desire for content or stuff and the form-drive as the means to manage that content (Bentley, 2009). Essential to Schiller's conceptualisation is his belief that there is a temporal dimension to the development of the three drives. The sense-drive comes first as awareness of sensation develops. Self-awareness then emerges as the form-drive and with it the ability to reason and rationalise. Finally, "only out of the interaction of both drives can the will be developed or freedom fostered"[18] and realised through the emergence of the play-drive. It is not until *Letter 20* that the aesthetic condition is described as a state of mind and then only in a footnote.[19] The inherent logic of Schiller's argument for the wholeness of personality is now conceived as a syllogistic pattern of changing behaviour over time:[20]

1. Beauty resides in wholeness as the full realisation of the sense and form drives (*Letters 11 to 15*).
2. Wholeness as the full realisation of the sense and form drives resides in freedom (as defined in *Letter 19*).
3. Therefore beauty resides in freedom (adapted from Beiser, 2005: 153).

Of course this is a state of mind, a transitory moment of awareness that now might be called an aesthetic experience. What Schiller proposes is not simply art appreciation, an ability to recognise the beautiful but something deeper, ephemeral and transcendent. And with its recognition comes an inner peace, a freedom to enjoy the moment whatever the circumstance, a uniquely human experience. My little cat lying in the sun beside me on the window sill as I write feels contentment from the warmth and my proximity but she probably has no sense of the aesthetic or awareness of a beautiful moment. So the essence of Schiller's contention is that what we understand as beauty in the appreciation of art objects is not the same as an *aesthetic experience* in his intended sense of beauty. In the latter there is a moment of complete co-ordination between form and content, between shape and feeling. It is not simply to enjoy the spectacle of a beautiful object as contemporary interpretations would have us believe but it is to have a heightened sense of awareness that is fleeting, momentary. In such moments there is a recognition of the integration of the individual with society, a sense of wholeness through the synthesis of contemplation and activity.[21] Jane has underlined a passage which suggests the features of aesthetic experience are "sensibility refined, feeling quickened, imagination enriched, and understanding enlarged".[22] In a slightly later work, Wilkinson and Willoughby further develop their analysis of the *Aesthetic Letters* in an explanation of Schiller's concept of the whole man achieved through and by aesthetic education. They suggest that the test Schiller proposes "for the genuineness of an aesthetic experience is that it should return us to the flux of life ready to meet whatever challenge presents itself, not more inclined to one mode of activity rather than another" (Wilkinson & Willoughby, 2002: 255).

While Schiller was writing the *Aesthetic Letters*, he was asked by his publisher, Cotta, to review a recently published pocket gardening calendar (Benn, 1991). This proved to be a fortuitous request as Schiller was able to use the review as a vehicle for his concept of the ideal garden. It is clear from his correspondence with Goethe (Schmitz, 1877) that having a garden was particularly important to Schiller for his own health and that of his family. In 1797 he purchased a garden house in Jena which he used as a summer retreat. The Cotta review is rarely considered in its own right but it does provide an empirical example for his theory of aesthetic education. Schiller contrasts the regular, geometric features of French gardens with the lawless freedom found in English gardens. The solution lies, of course, in the middle (third) way of German, landscaped gardens which "would appeal in equal measure to both the intellect and the emotions" (Benn, 1991: 32). In the review, Schiller uses the palace gardens at Hohenheim as an example of a landscaped place that is

> capable of leading the simple man to thought and the man of culture to feeling [that he regards] as a beautiful art form which is instrumental in bringing the opposing forces in man's psyche into a harmonious equilibrium and hence in furthering the aesthetic education of mankind.
>
> *(Benn, 1991: 40)*

In the *Aesthetic Letters* Schiller proposes art as key to the reintegration of man's alienation with modernity and his own inner conflicts without losing the benefits of sophistication (Sharpe, 1991). Yet this had only seemed achievable through the abstraction of beauty as an art form, such as the appreciation of classical Greek sculpture. Now, in a minor work on gardening, does his theory find practical application. However, while Schiller was known to have enjoyed walking and living in the countryside (Benn, 1991) he used the word 'nature' to refer not to "the phenomena themselves but the phenomena regarded as part of an abstract notion of nature's completeness and regularity, as well as of its innocence, perfection and harmony" (Sharpe, 1991: 177). In other words, it is in the synthesis of the natural landscape with human design that Schiller finds "the qualities which the ideal landscape garden must possess if it is to have an aesthetic effect on man" (Benn, 1991: 29).

A final point regarding Schiller is about his own health. In 1791 he suffered a possible "tubercular empyema of one lung that ruptured though his diaphragm into his abdominal cavity" (Bentley, 2009: 280). He was never well again and each winter expected to die from further serious illness. His continuing ill health gave him time to devote to his interest on aesthetic matters. However, pressure of work at the University of Jena and commitments to publishers led to anxiety that compounded his fragile state. In his later correspondence to the end of his life "we read time and again that cramps, breathlessness and numerous other physical discomforts have kept him from work. One frequently has the sense of someone kept alive by sheer force of will-power" (Sharpe, 1991: 119). This knowledge adds both a poignancy and a sense of the remarkable achievement of his efforts. It may also to some extent explain his particular interest in the aesthetic and tragedy thereby enhancing its value in this context.

Goethe's scientific studies

Despite his ill health and consequent financial difficulties, Schiller had many supporters. Goethe especially was in contact through letters and visits on an almost daily basis (Bentley, 2009) until Schiller's death. Goethe is credited with the shift in Schiller's thinking away from Kantian dualism of nature versus freedom, forcing him to reconsider his concept of wholeness. In Goethe, Schiller saw a man who was a well-rounded and fully integrated person, the perfect dynamic embodiment of his personality theory (Wilkinson & Willoughby, 1967). But Schiller had to acknowledge that for Goethe "the ideal of wholeness was only to be achieved as a changing pattern in time"[23] and not the static state of his initial conception. Unlike Schiller who relied on abstract ideas and notions to shape his theories, Goethe preferred to start from the close observation of a particular phenomenon to build an understanding of the whole (Sharpe, 1991).

Goethe's approach to science was through the eyes of the artist who saw an aesthetically pleasing work of art as one which "re-presents traces of lived experience in the meaningfully interconnected array of the textured surface of its physical medium, whether in paint or marble, in the sound and look of language, or in the undulating figurations of the dancer's body" (Stephenson,[24] 2005: 563). He was at odds with his contemporary scientific community and disliked mathematics, mechanics and astronomy which relied on a "system of quantitative signs [that] cannot adequately represent what we know qualitatively through experience" (Williams, 1998: 259). When Jane and I first met and she described her research and understanding of binary synthesis, I became interested in Goethean science. In particular the interpretation of Goethe's scientific studies of nature where "Goethe's mode of understanding sees the part in light of the whole, fostering a way of science which dwells in nature" (Bortoft, 1996: 4). Yet making sense of Goethe's scientific method and its relationship to binary synthesis, has presented something of a challenge not least because of the different interpretations of the source materials. As the original works were written in German either a comprehensive knowledge of the language is needed or an accurate translation. His scientific work has either been largely ignored as with the German-speaking world, or has been muddied by some exponents of 'Goethean science' who "draw on Rudolf Steiner, one of the earliest editors of Goethe's natural-scientific writings (yet, because of his status as the founding father of anthroposophy, something of a bugbear for many scholars)" (Bishop, 2015: 83). For me there are two specific difficulties: the tendency of those familiar with German to use untranslated quotations and with regard to Goethe's scientific writings, some interpretations of translated works.

To address these issues of translation and interpretation, my approach has been to work first from the translators or Germanists' accounts and explanations (Wilkinson & Willoughby, 1967; Sharpe, 1991; Stephenson, 2005), and then move to more interpretative accounts (Bortoft, 1996; Seamon, 1998; Zajonc, 1998; Wahl, 2005). Goethe's scientific method is not a precise set of steps to follow but a way of doing science that involves "heightened methodological awareness and sensitivity to the way we engage in the phenomenal world" (Holdrege, 2005: 27). Yet others cannot resist reducing the complexity by step-wise refinement (Wahl, 2005). A topic of Goethe's early discussions with Schiller was his idea of a primal plant or *Urpflanze* "which he insisted he could actually see in all individual plants" (Reed, 2002: 102). Schiller was unimpressed and remarked "it was a fine idea, but an idea, not an experience" (Williams, 1998: 266). Initially it had appeared that the two lacked any common ground but something sparked their interest in each other. They came to see themselves as "the contrasting halves of an ideal human and poetic wholeness" (Reed, 2002: 103); a living binary synthesis where the concepts from each would engage in an interplay of subordination and reciprocation. While Reed (2002) recounts their mutual influences in their dramatic and poetic works, Williams (1998) credits Schiller with encouraging Goethe to be more methodical in his scientific studies by including theory to balance his observations and experiences. Goethe's interests were not confined to his search for a primal plant but included all of the life sciences, which he termed morphology or the study of form. A development of this idea can be found in work on semantic category recognition or why a Labrador dog is 'doggier' than a Dachshund (Rosch, 1987).

Goethe was a passionate scientist for whom research was an ongoing mediation between direct experience and the tradition of the researcher (Steuer, 2002). In the context of this study, his most relevant scientific work is the *Zur Farbenlehre* or *Theory of Colour* first published in 1810 (Goethe, 1970). Goethe had attempted to refute Newton's colour theory, an exercise which proved to be ill-fated (Williams, 1998). However, it is his use of metaphorical language, cautioning against the use of signs for phenomena (Steuer, 2002) while seeing with the mind's eye, as the scientist's observations (Stephenson, 2005) that is apposite here. Part of the continuing attraction of the text is not the discredited theory, although there is some more recent evidence in its support (Zajonc, 1998) but the manner in which unorthodox ideas are presented. His purpose is to induce in the reader "a state of mind in which thought and perception become one" (Stephenson, 2005: 571). When this state occurs, the *Urphenomenon*, which can be understood as the primal phenomenon, appears (Bortoft, 1996; Seamon, 1998). Something he had been searching for in his earlier plant studies, Goethe now found through his understanding of colour. Essentially, he realised that there is a reciprocal relationship between light and darkness; without darkness, light cannot be perceived. From this interaction colours emerge as Goethe enthuses in the Preface to his Theory of Colours:

> Colours are the actions of light, actions and sufferings. In this sense, we can expect to learn about light from them. Colours and lights stand in the most precise relationship to one another; but we must think of both as belonging to the whole of Nature for it is she, as a whole, who wants to reveal herself concretely in this way to the sense organ of the eye. In exactly the same way Nature as a whole uncovers herself to every other sense. Close your eyes, prick up your ears and from the softest sound to the wildest noise, from the simplest tone to the highest harmony, from the most violent, passionate scream to the gentlest words of sweet reason, it is but Nature who speaks, revealing her being, her power, her life, and her relatedness so that a blind person, to whom the infinitely visible world is denied, can grasp an infinite vitality in what can be heard.
>
> *(Stephenson, 1995: 49–50)*

Beautiful as this passage is, it is also indicative of why such powerful prose might disconcert Goethe's contemporary scientific community.

The point is not the correctness or otherwise of the theory but that the colours perceived in everyday experience can be understood as having "an intrinsic necessity and therefore are understandable in themselves" (Seamon, 2005: 96). The *Urphenomenon* is not an easy concept to grasp despite various interpretations (Heinemann, 1934; Bortoft, 1996; Seamon, 2005). Nevertheless, there is something curiously attractive to the theory which perhaps speaks to a basic human desire for wholeness. A few apparently random lines will be interpreted by the human brain into a recognisable form or Gestalt; a glimpse of someone passing in the street leads to their recognition. This phenomenon can be explained through the different functionality of the brain's right and left hemispheres (McGilchrist, 2012). Simplistically, the left hemisphere is concerned with 'what' as individual bits of information while the right hemisphere, preoccupied by context, relational experience and emotion, is concerned with 'how' and making something whole, again a Gestalt. Consequently until recently neuroscience was more interested in the overall functionality of the brain and not the individual function of each hemisphere. Now the role of the right hemisphere is recognised as it delivers the new as "the primacy of experience" (McGilchrist, 2012: 179) while the left hemisphere re-presents what has been seen. This discussion of cerebral neuroscience may seem irrelevant but the connection lies with how Goethe's nineteenth-century concept of the *Urphenomenon* continues to inspire modern thought and interpretations.

Aesthetic discourse

Despite my efforts during the doctoral research to grasp Jane's understanding of binary synthesis, I knew there were some aspects that remained vague and unclear.

In addition to her fondness for the notion of the return enhanced, she often used the term 'import' in the sense of what I took to mean significance. But her use was in the sense of the word as translated from the eighteenth-century German, *Gehalt*, when it has a richer, deeper meaning. The term is especially relevant as a central concept in the aesthetics of Goethe and Schiller. Any work of art, including music, must have a content (*Gehalt*) but the materials (*Stoff*) used to make the form (*Gestalt*) "may or may not borrow the appearances of the world we know or follow the accepted rules of logic or even of syntax" (Wilkinson, 1959: 19). The difficulty now in understanding this distinction is compounded by the modern perception of content as simply what something is about. For Schiller the related term *Inhalt* is nearer to actual content and includes not just the raw materials of "clay or stone, paint and canvas, tones or language, but the forms of perception and experience – objects, persons, scenes and events – even cultural forms".[25] All of this content is broken down by the artist and assimilated through a process of metamorphosis into a new form. This is a *Gestalt* which has both the property of shape and also as described by Goethe "the whole complex of existence of an actual being".[26] Yet, in the aesthetic context, form is taken to a further level of abstraction with the inclusion of *Schein* or semblance as something coming into view. This term has the role of a master concept, the very essence of aesthetic experience, which for Schiller encompasses both a sense of shining and an illusory yet living quality. For both Goethe and Schiller, the concept is "some kind of illusion, and as something the artist creates, as a property of his work, not just as a way of looking at it, a quality which the appreciating mind projects into it" (Wilkinson, 1955: 223). An easy example from nature is a rainbow and from the arts, anything which has a 'felt life' as the true *Gehalt* of art.[27]

Goethe's scientific method had revealed the presence of the *Urphenomenon* through the study of individual forms – plants, rocks, rainbows – using a process of constant comparison between analysis and synthesis until the archetype or *Urphenomenon* appeared (Wilkinson & Willoughby, 1962). Yet Goethe was not comfortable in Schiller's world of abstraction, preferring sensuous embodiment by sketching the primal plant, "that essence of 'plantness'" (Wilkinson & Willoughby, 1962: 178) and using his preferred term, *Anschauung*, or "aesthetic perception"[28] (Stephenson, 1983: 65). The botanist Agnes Arber who had an interest in plant morphology and had translated Goethe's botanical writings (Wilkinson, 1948), interpreted his term *Anschauung* as one which combines "the intuitive knowledge gained through contemplation of the visible aspect" (Arber, 1950: 209). In turn, Schiller through his collaboration with Goethe had developed his theory of *schöner Vortrag*[29] or aesthetic discourse (Stephenson, 1995). This is where the "logical, conceptual relations and poetic structures in a text may be perceived as either coordinate with one another, or mutually subordinated to one another" (Plenderleith, 1993: 299). The purpose is to enable the reader to take the text as either communicative (it tells us something) or as poetic expression (we feel something from it) depending on the reader's need and capacity. However, if a complete fusion between the two modes occurs, the discursive prose then becomes poetry (Stephenson, 1983). Schiller's idea was that language used in such a way frees the psyche of the reader so clear reason can be brought into play. Stephenson (1983) has demonstrated how Goethe used Schiller's theory of aesthetic discourse in personal letters and in his *Maxims and Reflections*. For example:

> People say that between two opposed opinions truth lies in the middle.
> Not at all!
> A problem lies in-between, invisible, eternally active life, contemplated in peace.
> (Stephenson, 1983: 46 fn21)

In the German version (Stephenson, 1983: 176) the maxim is something of a tongue-twister and rich with alliteration for aesthetic appeal. The structure demonstrates the key to Schiller's theory where words or statements can be subordinate, co-ordinate or even super-ordinate to each other in reciprocal interplay (Wilkinson & Willoughby, 2002). Here the first sentence is deceptive suggesting truth can be found between two opinions and then subordinating it to the solution offered in the third sentence. But the relationship between the sentences creates a coordinate role revealing that what lies between the two statements produces a thought. And with this perceptible thought "the conceptual *distinction* becomes a felt *difference*" (Stephenson, 1983: 176). The tongue-twister contains a brain-twister – reason as understanding cooperates with the sense impression of aesthetic perception. What makes the maxim aesthetic is the co-ordination of abstract understanding "with what is presented to sense, as opposed to our ordinary, everyday, imaginative activity" (Stephenson, 1983: 162) where sense is subordinated to understanding. Aesthetic discourse then, in the Goethe–Schiller sense, has a distinctive feel and sound to it, not the rhythm of poetry, but nevertheless a pleasing quality. It is of course most apparent in the original German but it is also recognisable in translation. In Jane's doctoral work she examines Goethe's autobiography for the "relationship between 'poetry' and 'truth', between 'form' and 'meaning', in terms of its potential binary synthesis of the sacral realm of religious speculation and the secular context of the written word" (Plenderleith, 1993: 299). In her analysis she finds Goethe does not exploit religious material but makes "a positive affirmation of the sacral, enhanced as it is by a particular kind of inclusion in the secular context" (Plenderleith, 1993: 299).

It has been necessary, for the reasons given previously, to make a long and perhaps confusing journey through the complexities of Goethe and Schiller's philosophical ideas and language. Unravelling the nuanced meaning of German terms which had particular meanings for both men, though not necessarily the same, has also been somewhat challenging. Now a connection can be made to aesthetic experience from the emergence of binary synthesis in Schiller's *Aesthetic Letters* with Goethe's scientific philosophy of the *Urphenomenon*.

Binary synthesis and the return enhanced

Notwithstanding all of the detailed descriptions of Goethe and Schiller's philosophical efforts, neither them of course either used or had any idea of the term *binary synthesis*. It originated, as stated earlier in the chapter, with Wilkinson and Willoughby, the most scholarly of the translators of the *Aesthetic Letters*. They further refine their analysis to demonstrate the process of progressive intensification and refinement or *Steigerung*. This is attributed to Goethe's[30] scientific studies and Stephenson later translates the term as "upward enhancement" (1995: 13) which is nearer to my recollection of Jane's understanding. The interplay between each pair of polarised concepts reveals not the discovery of a new condition to improve human nature but on the better use of those already possessed. Jane has underlined the key passage and used square brackets for further emphasis, where binary synthesis is defined as the return enhanced:

> And by raising, now the one, now the other antithesis to the synthesis he can express his belief that [the return is in reality a progress]: that by trying to discover what man's true nature is, we shall at the same time discover the destination towards which he should go.[31]

While Jane did not actually publish her understanding of the return enhanced, she did provide her own interpretation of binary synthesis:

> The most arresting and stimulating aspect of such a synthesis is perhaps that it is not logical (in the sense that logic is a mode of thought based on conceptual implication). Binary synthesis is descriptive of the process of existence rather than prescriptive of the process of logic. The oppositions in a binary synthesis function truly only together, but they remain distinct: either or both of the fundamental polarities appears enhanced through reciprocal, subordinating interaction with the other.
>
> (Plenderleith, 1993: 298)

Despite the very detailed explanations of Wilkinson and Willoughby, and my subsequent interpretations the actual point of all of this aesthetic education may remain unclear. To reiterate, my purpose was to try and understand what I believed Jane understood of an obscure and largely ignored aspect of German Idealism. Certainly this is not a concept which has reached a wider audience. The highly specialised world of a few German scholars, mostly connected by the supervision of doctoral theses, has all the feel and dark shadows of the garret in an ivory tower. But what do I now take forward from this into the next chapters and carry to the final conclusions? What can now be understood from Schiller's *Aesthetic Letters* is the emergence of binary synthesis as a complex communication style for philosophical ideas that emphasise the necessity for man's holistic well-being of aesthetic experience. This is aesthetic discourse (*schöner Vortrag*), the reciprocal interplay of aesthetic and logical language which can be either communicative or expressive. From Goethe comes an equally philosophical yet more practical view of nature as an observable whole which first necessitates the complete knowledge of the phenomena that is then made one's own through reflection. In a little essay on polarity, Goethe sets out the circular process of moving from the particular to the general and then the return (enhanced) to the particular:

> Duality of the phenomenon as opposites:
> We and the objects
> Light and dark
> Body and soul
> Two souls
> Spirit and matter
> God and world
> Thought and extension
> Ideal and real
> Sensuality and reason
> Fantasy and practical thought
> Being and yearning
> Two halves of the body
> Right and left
> Breathing.
> Physical experiment:
> Magnet.
>
> (Goethe, 2016: 951)

In the commentary below the poem, just in case the reader has not quite grasped his point, Goethe goes on to explain:

> Whatever appears in the world must divide if it is to appear at all. What has been divided seeks itself again, can return to itself and reunite. This happens in a lower sense when it merely intermingles with its opposite, combines with it; here the phenomenon is nullified or at least neutralised. However, the union may occur in a higher sense if what has been divided is first intensified; then in the union of the intensified halves it will produce a third thing, something newer, higher, unexpected.
>
> (Goethe, 2016: 951)

Earlier Goethe's concept of *Anschauung* or aesthetic perception was introduced as a way to sense the appearance of an *Urphenomenon*. This is the aesthetic experience of reality in all its elemental dynamism, revealed as a world ordered by the rhythmic patterns at work within us and felt as a rising tension that intensifies and then resolves (Stephenson, 1995). By now the earlier description of the return enhanced as a way of recognising something that had perhaps been experienced previously but not then fully appreciated can be understood as a great simplification of some very complex processes. At the heart of this interplay is binary synthesis which for Schiller results in something new as a product of two other concepts whilst for Goethe it is the intense recognition of something anew as its very essence.

Part three: research aesthetics

The final part of this chapter outlines some aspects of the approaches used in the study and an overview of the specifically developed self-directed interview method. Underpinning the research was an ethical framework designed to address from the outset the obvious potential ethical issues: the subject was deceased, the researcher was their partner and there is no tangible evidence of consent. Taking an open and honest stance from the beginning was indicative of a genuine concern that the study should be consistently ethically grounded. Ethical awareness was ensured by using continuous consent (Allmark et al., 2009) where those engaged in the research reaffirm their commitment to continue. This did not just apply to the self-directed interviews but also to my own relationship with the study. There were occasions when I did question the wisdom of continuing with the personal nature of the study. The relationship between the experience of my partner's dying and the research methodology was a real struggle. I actively avoided committing to any particular approach believing that as the study was essentially a form of narrative inquiry (Riessman, 2008) the rest would follow when needed. But I was confusing narrative inquiry as a field of study (MacLaren, 2014) with the necessarily precise account of why and how the research was done. My resistance had many strands but centred on the role of the *Aesthetic Letters* and binary synthesis to the research. I could not reconcile my 'felt-sense' (Gendlin, 2004) that the approach must have something to do with this obscure methodological tool. Yet I was also aware that the study could not be driven by some intellectual whim or trying to emulate Jane's doctoral work.

The resolution to the tension between what I wanted to study and how it could be done was found by tracing a convoluted path forward through the human sciences to a phenomenology of practice (van Manen, 2014) and then back through the later philosophy of Heidegger to Goethe and binary synthesis. The approach used here had many influences but the focus was sharpened by Heidegger's distinction between contemplative thinking as receptive yet meditative awareness, and calculative thinking that is "'always on the move' and merely 'doing' an existing pattern of organized thought" (Galvin & Todres, 2007: 39). This 'letting be' opens up creative possibilities for "feeling, thinking and doing" (Galvin & Todres, 2007: 33) as a seamless integration of heart, head and hand. Viewed in this way, the doctoral research design integrated the desire to act in the right way (heart) in consideration of the underlying philosophies (head) and appropriate action for the data collection and analysis (hand). The approach necessitated an ethical sensitivity both to the needs of those directly involved in the study (me, supervisors, interviewer) and a sense of heightened awareness towards the data field. Let me unpack this a little before proceeding to the actual account.

Goethe's idea of aesthetic perception or *Anschauung* was introduced earlier, but more recently *Anschauung* has been translated as 'aesthetic intuition' for any "instances of sensuous perception that occur within the open-ended, cyclical, process of ever more specific (and ever more theorized) insight" (Stephenson, 2005: 563).

While it is important to acknowledge that the term has a precise meaning in the context of Goethe's scientific and literary methods, it might also be in a very similar place to Gendlin's concept of a 'felt sense' where experience is "a process of carrying forward, occurring into implying, reaching back behind itself in going forward" (Gendlin, 2004: 146). And while this description has a flavour of *Anschauung*, Gendlin draws on neither Goethe nor Schiller in his explication of a psychotherapeutic approach based on recognising an implicit bodily awareness where "what comes in this way feels more deeply and uncensoredly from yourself, than anything that you could construct" (Gendlin, 2004: 132). But there was something familiar to me in this description as I wrote the doctoral dissertation when I needed a connection between the return enhanced as an interplay between the knowledge insights from the literature and how this felt in relation to the study.

I came to understand these feelings as a kind of 'aesthetic phenomenology where there is "a concern to portray the lived 'sensuous taste' of what an experience may be and feel like" (Galvin & Todres, 2011: 525). When this approach is used to report research findings, it has "the potential to transform the reader or audience in ways that good poetry does, in that it can move or touch us" (Galvin & Todres, 2011: 525). It seemed important that the thesis, as the principal product of the original study, was engaging to read. For this reason, the narrative account of *The Illness Period* is located nearer to the genre of fictional illness writing for its textural insights than narrative inquiry as a structuring device. In this way the direction of inquiry can be viewed as being towards a narrative purpose that gathers experiential accounts. It is actually immensely difficult to describe the writing process in formal research terms. I cannot put into words what I did with the various textual sources that are the basis to the illness narrative. But what I can do is say a little more about the fictional and other works that helped along the way. This explanation is as an alternative to presenting the methodology of the study as given in the thesis (Adamson, 2015) as what really mattered then and now is not what I actually did but how I felt my way through the texts. And it is only now, with all it means to return enhanced, that I can see the process as one of aesthetic intuition with its felt sense and increasing insight – every return adds another moment of meaning.

Writing illness

Fictional writing about illness, disease and dying has within its genre well-known works such as Aleksandr Solzhenitsyn's *Cancer Ward* (1970) and Gabriel García Márquez' *Love in the Time of Cholera* (1988). Both were preceded by the real masterwork (Byatt, 2005), Thomas Mann's *The Magic Mountain* (2005), with the first English translation published in 1928. In essence the story is a protracted account over seven years of a young man's experience of tuberculosis and his extended stay in a Swiss sanatorium. Appropriately, for the context here, Mann draws on Goethe in three distinct ways: first the novel is essentially pedagogical, a Bildungsroman intended to educate the central character, Hans Castorp, and follows a similar path to Goethe's own Bildungsroman, *Wilhelm Meister* (Gesler, 2000). Second, one character, the scholar Herr Settembrini, makes regular quotations from Faust (Byatt, 2005). Finally, while writing the text and then within it, Mann drew heavily on Goethean science, integrating a compendium of scientific ideas from that time (Greenberg, 1985). Read in this way, a central theme of *The Magic Mountain* is the inextricable link between art and science, beauty and nature. Mann's real achievement in the book is the way he plays with the nature of disease and its brutal realities in contrast with the positive aspects of disease and death as spiritual insights (Gesler, 2000). In this last aspect, Mann makes a firm connection back to German Romanticism and therefore Goethe's literary work. In other political writings, Mann makes use of binary synthesis in a similar fashion to its first use by Goethe and Schiller (Bishop, 2005).

A bridge from fictional writing about illness to non-fiction can be found in works such as Virginia Woolf's *On Being Ill* and her mother, Julia Stephen's, *Notes from a Sick Room* (Woolf, 2012). The daughter writes of illness obliquely, as an aesthetic project that attempts to render the otherwise linearity of illness, as simultaneously "a heightened state of awareness that cannot be learned, perfected, or replicated by another" (Coates, 2012: 9). Woolf's essay repudiates Stephen's emphasis on the 'art of nursing' in favour of the 'art of being ill' where illness is privileged with a vantage point from which to view the world (Coates, 2012). More recent illness writing may have lost some of Woolf's deep, philosophical insights but it is now a burgeoning field. Book length accounts of illness are rare before the 1900s and uncommon until after 1950 (Hawkins, 1993). Then from the 1960s onwards there is a steady rise in pathographies, "a form of autobiography or biography that describes personal experience of illness, treatment and sometimes both" (Hawkins, 1993: 1). Within this genre, if works are categorised by authorial intent, early examples are largely testimonies to the strength of the sufferer and their positive disposition towards the medical profession. Towards the end of the 1970s there is a dramatic change and a split into two distinct and opposing types of pathography. In the first, the authorial intent comes from "a sense of outrage over particular and concrete instances of what is perceived to be the failure of medicine to care adequately for the ill" (Hawkins, 1993: 6). In contrast, the second type is less at odds with the vagaries of modern medicine and speaks to "a patient population empowered by a belief in the near limitless capacities of the mind and the emotions to facilitate healing" (Hawkins, 1993: 9). Whatever the type, the purpose of these narratives is twofold: heroic recognition in the battle against either disease and/or the medical profession, and as an intentionally helpful travel guide through the strange and unfamiliar landscape of illness.

During the research, possibly from reading too much Goethe and Schiller (can there be such a state), I gave serious consideration to a fictionalised account of *The Illness Period*. It seemed to offer certain advantages, not least the avoidance of ethical concerns over anonymity and confidentiality. But to me the narrative would just be yet another story lacking the embodied authenticity of the real account. Before me were piles (literal, metaphorical and digital) of text but despite knowing the story inside out, upside down and back to front, I just did not know where or even how to begin. Should it be with a potted biography of Jane's childhood, university days and myriad events before I knew her? Certainly a story but not of her illness and death. I needed to determine the temporal and spatial boundaries or I would just wander aimlessly through second-hand memories. Locating these edges was essential for deciding what lay within the diffuse landscape of the study and equally what remained beyond its boundary. Inevitably some of the edges were fuzzy, eroded by particular tensions leaving them barely discernible. Yet it was at these edges that important insights occurred. Feeling for these edges and letting them arise naturally from within allows meaning to move from being constructed to being embodied. Writing illness in this 'felt-sense' (Gendlin, 2004) accords with aesthetic phenomenology as 'embodied relational understanding' (Todres, 2008).

> Embodied relational understanding refers to a way of knowing that is holistically contextual, that is, a form of knowledge that is attentive to the rich and moving flow of individuals lives in relation to others, is attentive to very specific situations, and to the inner worlds of what it is like for patients to 'go through something'.
>
> *(Galvin & Todres, 2011: 523)*

Conventionally studies of cancer and palliative care experiences for both patients and carers have relied primarily but not exclusively on interviews (Thomas, 2009; Jack & O'Brien, 2010; Kendall et al., 2010; Payne, 2010) or diaries (Campion-Smith et al., 2011). A defining characteristic of this group is that they are all researcher-led. The studies set out to answer a specific question about the nature of the experience of the sufferer and, where included, their primary carer. Other studies have capitalised on existing narratives, particularly blogs (Bingley et al., 2006; Heilferty, 2009; Kim, 2009; O'Brien & Clark, 2010). In this group, the person with the illness experience is the initiator of the narrative, normally with therapeutic or existential purposes (Bingley et al., 2006). Psychological studies that use standard questionnaire instruments to gauge anxiety or some other measurable feature of the person's experience (see George 2002; Yao et al., 2007) were discounted as not being pertinent to an understanding of everyday life in a social context.

The clearly definable start and end points delineated by diagnosis and death established the temporal boundaries. But there are other boundaries here. Langellier (2003) sees personal narrative as a liminal or boundary state, a place of transition between the personal and the public. Froggatt (1997) extends the concept of liminality in her study of hospice work, finding it a state of transition for both the dying and the bereaved. Both views are relevant here. There are boundaries around what can be shared for public consumption and the boundary of the shared experience. The related concepts of boundedness as bodily deterioration (Lawton 1998) and the forced embodiment of sickness (Skott, 2002) may also be pertinent. Having considered some interpretations and configurations of the boundaries that might be relevant, the need to make sense of what had happened as a whole, from the beginning (diagnosis) to the end (death) became apparent. This could be resolved using a sequence of time-ordered stories connected by a process of inquiry through writing (Richardson, 2000), that would lead to understanding.

Boundaries can also help to determine meaning. According to Heidegger, we are practically engaged with our lifeworld through sensation and in such a way that any encounter comes with meaning and significance (van Manen, 2007). For example, looking at a timepiece it is not simply an optical sensation but usually involves a question 'how long until lunch?' or 'when will …?'. It is therefore in the "context of meaning in which our practices are embedded" (van Manen, 2007). We understand the world through our own way of being in the world which is informed by our cultural understandings and experiences. Heidegger's perspective is ontological, a theory of being. It connects with the human desire to see living form as part of a greater whole, as a movement towards "coming into-Being" (Shotter, 2000: 234). Drawing on Goethe's phenomenological methods, this living form can be interpreted as one which,

> instead of seeking to explain a present activity in terms of the past, we can understand … in terms of its meaning for us, that is, in terms of our spontaneous responses to it. It is only from within our involvements with other living things that this kind of meaningful, responsive understanding becomes available to us.
>
> *(Shotter, 2000: 234)*

It can be argued that a holistic understanding of narrative is one that conflates both ontology and epistemology, as a theory of knowledge, with no discernible space between knowledge and action (Butler-Kisber, 2010). This accords with Goethe's view from his Bildungsroman, *Wilhelm Meister* first published in 1821:[32]

> Thinking and doing, doing and thinking, that is the sum total of all wisdom, recognised of old, practised of old, not realised by everybody. Like breathing in and breathing out, both are eternally moving backwards and forwards in perpetual motion: like question and answer, the one cannot really happen without the other.

These apparent polar opposites of thinking and doing can only make sense in relation to one another, especially in a narrative context; without one, the other fails to function. The implied rhythm also has a tempo, a timeline along which the interplay occurs, a narrative thread. Stanley, in her study of biography, defines the Bildungsroman as the autobiographical archetype "the tale of the progressive travelling of a life from troubled or stifled beginnings; in which obstacles are overcome and the true self actualised or revealed" (Stanley, 1992: 11). Returning to insights from German literature provides a contrasting definition of Bildungsroman where "issues are framed less in terms of practicality (of which the realist novel speaks) than with a view to a philosophically differentiated definition and exploration of the interplay of self and world" (Swales, 2002: 143).

While others have claimed their doctoral dissertations are themselves Bildungsroman (Jacobs, 2008; Knowles & Promislow, 2008), there was no attempt to do something similar but the genre did help to inform the underlying philosophy driving the research. In an ontological-epistemological sense the study was the analytic account of troubled lives where obstacles are overcome and the authentic self (of the carer/researcher/writer) becomes actualised. Liz Stanley kept a research diary as an exercise in 'intellectual autobiography' where she explored her attempts to make sense of her mother's self, following a stroke and summarises the process thus:

> I have also used these diary extracts to construct a narrative – to 'tell a story' – around a set of ontological problematics (what did all this mean, regarding my mother's self, regarding myself, regarding selves and consciousness in general) with epistemological consequentiality (what did all this entail for how I, we, understand what it is to have knowledge about another person, about one's self).
>
> (Stanley, 1993: 211)

The act of writing is in itself transformative just as the narration by clients as processes of remembering and retelling are key elements in counselling and psychotherapy conversations (Riessman & Speedy, 2007). There is no single, true meaning to be found within this study. There are as many meanings, understandings and interpretations as there are readers; each will see it as part of a greater whole as it comes into being.

Narrative inquiry

Although drawn to more fictionalised accounts of illness narratives, I also explored and utilised aspects of narrative inquiry. Story telling is a defining characteristic of human behaviour; no other mammal has the language to tell stories. Stories imbue all aspects of our lives from the very private inner workings of the stories we tell ourselves to the public accounts of our behaviour and actions. The idea of using narrative in the social sciences began in the 1960s, gathering momentum to the extent that it is now everywhere, in every discipline, every profession (Riessman & Speedy, 2007).

Framing research as narrative has been defined as allowing the researcher "to see different and sometimes contradictory layers of meaning, to bring them into useful dialogue with each other, and to understand more about individual and social change" (Squire et al., 2008: 1). But what is narrative itself and is it synonymous with story? The linguistic origins are different and therefore give some clue to more nuanced interpretations. The word *narrative* is a compound adjective or noun from narrate plus the suffix -ive, both derived from the Latin, *gnarus* or knowing with a descriptive quality or nature (*SOED*, 2007) while story is also from Latin, *historia* – history. As Frank has commented, the terms are often used interchangeably yet "people do not tell narratives, they tell stories" (Frank, 2000: 354).

Riessman and Speedy distinguish narrative from other forms of discourse through the use of sequence and consequence within the narrative structure where "Events are selected, organized, connected, and evaluated as meaningful for a particular audience" (Riessman & Speedy, 2007: 430). However, both story and discourse can be seen as elements of narrative and can include the action of telling. In this configuration, a story is an abstract sequence of events while discourse is text in a particular medium or form, and telling is the act of narrating that produces the story (Bruner, 1986).

In general terms, researchers who engage in narrative inquiry find no difficulty in distinguishing between the phenomenon that is the story and the act of inquiry as the narrative, as "people by nature lead storied lives and tell stories of those lives, whereas narrative researchers describe such lives, collect and tell stories of them, and write narratives of experience" (Connelly & Clandinin, 1990: 2). However, this clarity may have become smudged as it has been suggested that there is a fault-line which "concerns 'narrative studies' (signalling a focus on narrative as a particular kind of data or the content of this) as compared with 'narrative inquiry' (signalling narrative as a methodological and analytical approach by the researcher)" (Stanley & Temple, 2008: 276). Definitions of narrative inquiry are likely to be dependent on the parent discipline with nuanced different positions between sociologists, psychologists and educationalists. A simple interpretation that resonated with the study is "narrative inquiry is a way of understanding experience" (Clandinin & Connelly 2000: 20). Their approach centres on the collection of 'field texts' which are 'composed' and are what "passes for data in narrative inquiry" (Clandinin & Connelly 2000: 93). These texts can range from existing artefacts and include journal entries, field notes and research interview transcripts. Analysis is facilitated by appropriate archival processes to store the field texts, usually in chronological order.

Once the field texts are in order, an iterative process is used as the researcher-writer shuttles back and forth, weaving the emergent research text into a cloth that can be shaped and tailored through editing to fit the intended purpose. The energy and enthusiasm for narrative inquiry, and the eagerness to engage with its complex and nuanced storied experiences is compelling (Clandinin & Rosiek, 2007). Despite the difficulties of writing in this way, narrative inquiry is seductive in its prospect of novel and innovative possibilities. There is nothing inherently wrong with more conventional approaches that examine through thematic analysis 'what' is said in the content of a story, and through structural analysis 'how' it is said or organised (Riessman 2008). Yet even when told in this way, these stories continue to speak to us (van Manen, 2006), to find their real meaning (Sharp, 1996) perhaps hoping to become 'thrice told tales' (Riessman 2004). However, the inquirer needs to maintain a continual awareness of the interaction, continuity and situation within the narrative (Clandinin & Connelly, 2000). The researcher reading a text is simultaneously aware of three dimensions: the temporality of past, present and future; the interaction between people and events; and the place or space where the action is located. This sense of movement can now be carried forward to writing when "we may go back and forth a number of times until we get a feeling of aesthetic satisfaction that the words are good enough to carry forward the aliveness of the meanings" (Todres & Galvin, 2008: 577).

Recognising the serial nature of the narrative from *The Illness Period* as one which unfolds over time and has a chronological sequence, I turned to life story (Atkinson, 2007) and biographical interview methods (Jones, 2003; Bornat, 2008) to inform the approach to the self-directed interviews. Each method aims to capture an individual's life story but they differ in process and none address the issue of the known subject. Conventionally, research subjects or 'ordinary people' (Wengraf, 2000: 140) are recruited through third parties such as organisational settings or from somewhere the target group are known to congregate. Consequently, those who are co-opted to the study are unlikely to be known to the researcher; indeed if they are known they will be discounted by the study's exclusion criteria. This tradition is seen to have many benefits including the anonymity of the research subjects and conformity to ethical research standards. However, if the subject of the inquiry is no longer alive, how does that then alter and affect the position and rights within the narrative? In an autoethnographic context, loss is a prevalent topic and in particular the death of an intimate other (Ellis, 2007). If a relational view is included in the appraisal of the ethical dimensions of a study, then some of the potential difficulties that might arise, can be addressed. For example those who choose to write about personal loss feel that "our stories about people who have died serve as memorials that keep our loved ones alive in our memories" (Ellis, 2007: 14). But this feeling may not be shared by other family members. The research subject who can no longer respond or defend the representation of themselves is also likely to be a member of a family, a work colleague or an individual known to others. These relational others may not recognise the representation of the person being made by the researcher. While a deceased person may no longer enjoy the same legal rights as the living (Ellis, 2007), nevertheless there is a moral obligation on the researcher not just to be respectful but to be considerate of the others who knew the person concerned. Clearly, there is an assumption that the identity of the research subject is known and while "strategies such as fictionalising and blurring identities and places" (Clandinin & Huber, 2010: 439) may be used to conceal, it is perhaps better to minimise the risk of causing upset by honouring known sensitivities.

What is evident from any of the approaches to biographical interviews is that there are two roles involved, a research interviewer and a research subject, and they are not conflated. The interview participants may even be engaged in a conversation (Kvale, 2007) or in a novel, interactive process of discovery (Ellis et al., 2011). If the primary focus of the research is to explore a personal experience then the most common approach to capturing that testimony is simply to write it as a personal narrative (Langellier, 1999) or as an autoethnographic account (Ellis & Bochner, 2000; Ellis et al., 2011). Self-interview techniques were also investigated where respondents use a voice recorder to capture their reflections on a specific topic, possibly in response to a stimulus such as a photograph or artefact (Allett et al., 2011). This can be advantageous as it allows the self-interviewee to pause and reflect on their recollections and memories. But this self-reflection could also result in filtering by the respondent of difficult or sensitive areas in a manner similar to that suggested by Wengraf (2000) as motivation not to remember. If an interviewer is present, problematic areas can be explored within the constraints outlined above. Auto-interviewing (Boufoy-Bastick, 2004) which utilises similar techniques as those for self-interview was also explored. However, the purpose has a more anthropological slant as it attempts to surface culturally embedded worldviews of 'epic reporting' (Boufoy-Bastick, 2004: 3), a process which utilises the 'thick description' (Geertz, 1973) of visual memories. This approach was near to my purpose but the cultural focus was too broad. Realising there was no ideal method to elicit my recollections of *The Illness Period*, I decided to develop the self-directed interview method.

Documents of life

At the time of the original study it seemed important because of ethics and confidentiality to not use the actual dates of blog posts, email or hospital documents. Instead I just used the day number counting day one from when I noticed something was wrong to the last day when Jane died. But during the revisions for this book I have added some earlier blog posts to Chapter 2 and more time has passed. The artifice no longer seems necessary as it makes the time frame overly complicated. Using the actual date might help the reader to have a better sense of when things happened particularly as there are references to Christmas and other seasonal events. The temporal boundary as *The Illness Period* is defined as the time from a specific incident when it occurred to me that Jane might be seriously ill to her death. Existing calendars and diaries were used to create a spreadsheet time line as a chronological guide to the sequence of events during *The Illness Period*, a total of 342 days. In spatial terms, the location of all events is central Scotland but no details are given of specific personal places. The action is mainly in Edinburgh which may add a sense of aesthetic as it is a beautiful place.

In temporal terms, there were two types of field text: pre-existing documents from *The Illness Period* and the interview transcripts created during the study. The pre-existing documents were either personal materials written primarily by me or Jane, or official documents such as hospital letters. After the interviews started it became clear that some factual aspects of the recollections could, indeed should, be validated against the health records. The rationale was that an essential dimension to the overall story might be missed if the narrative account relied solely on personal documents. The justification and purpose was to verify the accuracy of events in the interview through reference to the historical account in the health records. However, gaining access to the health records took eight months of convoluted procedures. Records were held in two different hospitals as well as the general practitioner (GP) records. Despite all three care providers being within the same local health board and a unified ethical approval process, the reality was otherwise. Although access was applied for and granted by the NHS Research Ethics Committee, the primary care records required a different procedure. A further application had to be made to the practitioner services division within the health board. The decision to grant access was then passed to the GP practice who felt guidance was necessary from both the Medical Defence Union and the General Medical Council, despite the assurances provided by the various approvals and my lead supervisor. Once these sensitivities had been addressed, I was able to access all of Jane's health records. After conversion to digital format and cataloguing, the final corpus contained 175 field texts, organised both chronologically and by source against *The Illness Period* timeline. For the study, a process similar to the life history calendar (Freedman et al., 1988) was used where events are plotted over time.

Prior to deciding on third-party interviews, I had first tried to just write my recollections but I kept getting stuck and then veering off into polemic. Then I tried reclining on a couch with a digital recorder and rambled away but the results were similar. My concerns were about the rigour and appropriateness of interviewing myself as I tried to access the various stories of what had happened. I talked to a friend who has known me for many years and who is also a counsellor, about my sleepless nights of pondering the problem. What emerged was a mutual willingness to attempt a novel approach where we would conduct a series of interviews using an outline storyboard that I would provide. As I developed and refined the process, I thought in terms of two time periods, *then* when key events occurred, and *now* as those events are remembered.

My friend agreed to be the interviewer once she had sought professional guidance and support from her counselling supervisor. In turn I had permission first from my doctoral supervisors and then the necessary ethical approval. Given our personal friendship and to seal the agreement as a professional arrangement, an appropriate fee was remunerated. To clarify our roles and remit, and for the avoidance of doubt or ambiguity, a memorandum of understanding (MoU) was also used. The process of identifying, categorising and ordering the pre-existing field texts against the timeline had helped to identify the distinct episodes that would be the basis for each interview. The interviews were intended to each last approximately one hour and I calculated that if each storyboard had six cells with ten minutes' worth of material that would be sufficient for an interview. Storyboards are most commonly found in the creative industries where they give an overview of the scenes for a film, television show or advertisement and consist of a series of cells containing a visual depiction of each scene or frame (Cristiano, 2008). The field texts were reviewed for suitable extracts such as what was happening to Jane, or in general at particular times. The principal materials used were calendar events, blog posts and personal diary entries. For some storyboards short extracts from email correspondence and hospital discharge letters were used. Each storyboard covered a particular episode of variable length and each had a title drawn from either the field texts or my recollections.

Naming each episode had the immediate effect of framing its content. Once each storyboard was ready, it was sent to the interviewer for review and she then prepared her own schedule of questions. The purpose of the interviews was that while I was very familiar with the overall story, I wanted the interviews to capture the fine detail and 'thick description' (Geertz, 1973) of particular events and episodes. The core brief for the interviewer was to find out what I actually observed Jane feeling or experiencing. So although I effectively became the research subject, the interviewer's paraphrasing of the storyboard was to ease conversation and did not alter the intent of the inquiry. It was also important that I did not rehearse before an interview. Although I was clearly defining and bounding the topics for each interview, I wanted them to be fresh.

We met at the interviewer's counselling rooms as a neutral place and to avoid being disturbed, using the first interview to pilot the process. All went according to plan with some minor adjustments and the remaining ten interviews were conducted between August and November 2013. Each interview was recorded and then transcribed by me as at that time I did not want anyone else to hear the recordings. I also felt some familiarity with the text could be gained from the process despite its tedious nature. A tidy version of each transcript was extracted for analysis by taking Plummer's (2001: 150) recommendation to adopt Finnegan's approach; edit the transcript and remove hesitations, corrections, non-standard spellings and incorrect punctuation (Finnegan, 1992).

Once the corpus was complete and in digital format, it was organised into document types: blog posts, storyboards, medical records, and email. Fortuitously at this time, I heard the Irish author, Bernard MacLaverty on BBC Radio 4 talking about his literary life (Open Book, 2013). He recounted how a school teacher had asked him to summarise his stories into a single word. It occurred to me that this might be a useful way of scaffolding the narrative. I made a list of one word titles which were not the same as those used for the interview episodes. They can therefore be interpreted as indicative of a transition from the 'felt sense' of my experience to one of 'contemplative thinking' as a return enhanced. The single word title helped to keep in focus what each episode was about as it was being written. The narrative weaves between the two principal voices, mine from the interviews and Jane's from her blog posts, connected by an analytic thread. This does two things: first it makes the connections between the various texts and second, it turns to the literature to explain aspects of the story. This process illustrates the creative possibility, suggested earlier, of "feeling, thinking and doing" (Galvin & Todres, 2007: 33). The intention was the seamless integration of feeling my way into the texts, then thinking about possible explanations for particular aspects before doing the writing, a continual process of heart, head and hand. The first drafts made extensive use of both interview and blog extracts; I did not have the heart to reduce them. Gradually, the quotations were reduced as the essence of each was found and a sense of aesthetic phenomenology began to emerge. But the process is deeper, an embodied interpretation in the making. Gendlin (2004) describes a bodily process of a 'felt-sense' coming into language as words like sleep or tears and "what comes in this way feels more deeply and uncensoredly from yourself than anything that you could construct" (Gendlin, 2004: 132). This is in the same philosophical place as Heidegger's coming into Being which reaches back to Goethe and the *Urphenomenon*. It is abiding with the feeling of the experience and waiting for it to come into words that are often surprising but also have that immediate sense of being the right ones.

In this first chapter I have set the scene and context of the original study with its novel exploration of a witnessed personal account of a life limited by illness on which this book is based. Since the doctoral work, I have realised that the treatment of binary synthesis and the return enhanced in the thesis (Adamson, 2015) was insufficient to grasp Jane's deep understanding of these particular aspects of eighteenth-century German philosophy. Consequently in this chapter I have provided a more detailed account of both Schiller's theory of aesthetic education and Goethe's conceptual understanding of natural phenomena. Some German terms with their nuanced meaning in an eighteenth-century context have been introduced as they were part of Jane's everyday language. In particular, the return enhanced as the process of binary synthesis as well as import or the real significance of something are highlighted. The next three chapters provide the account of Jane's illness, from diagnosis to death. Occurrences which appear to have the qualities of an aesthetic experience as set out above will be highlighted. In the final chapter, the central themes of the return enhanced and aesthetic experience will be revisited to confirm my belief that these concepts provided Jane with the spiritual foundation from which she could understand and endure the vicissitudes of her illness.

Notes

1 The word 'man' here is translated from the German 'Menschen' or human being and not simply a male person.
2 Edited and Translated, with an Introduction, Commentary and Glossary of Terms. Henceforth quotations are footnoted and abbreviated to WW (Plenderleith, 1991: 13) and citations as Wilkinson & Willoughby (1967).
3 See Chapter 3: Treating.
4 Johann Gottlieb Fichte (1762–1814) professor of philosophy at the University of Jena.
5 "[T]he famous 'birthday letter'" (Sharpe, 1991: 142).
6 The name Kallias is derived from the Greek *kallos* meaning beauty.
7 Schaper (1985: 154) defines *Aesthetic Letters* as the usual abbreviation for the full title.
8 WW: xi.
9 WW: 1.
10 There is now a new translation by Keith Tribe (Schiller, 2016).
11 I use the term psyche in the same fashion as Hunt "to denote the complex mind, including both the conscious and unconscious mental processes, and sense of self" (2013: 28 fn1).
12 WW: lxxxv.
13 WW: li.
14 WW: li.
15 WW: 79.
16 WW: 105.
17 WW: 123.
18 WW: xcii.
19 WW: 141.
20 WW: lxxxiv.
21 WW: lxxxiv.
22 WW: lxxxv.

23 WW: xxxix.
24 There is a serendipitous trinity here with the introduction of Roger Stephenson, Emeritus Professor of German, University of Glasgow who was Jane's doctoral supervisor. His supervisor was Professor Elizabeth Wilkinson, University College London, co-editor and translator of the *Aesthetic Letters*.
25 WW: 318.
26 WW: 309.
27 WW: 310.
28 Wilkinson and Willoughby, suggest "intuitive contemplation" (1962: 177) which illustrates both the difficulty of translation and the nuanced meaning.
29 WW: cxviii.
30 WW: xciv.
31 WW: lxxxvi – square brackets as added by Jane.
32 This translation is from Jane's personal papers. Perhaps academia is inclined to fall into a Cartesian trap in its desire to separate ontology from epistemology; one cannot really exist, even in a philosophical sense, without the other.

References

Adamson, Veronica (1999) *Shifting Paradigms*, Dissertation (MEd), Department of Adult and Continuing Education: University of Sheffield

Adamson, Veronica (2015) *The Dance to Death: The Aesthetic Experience of Dying*, PhD Thesis, Edinburgh: University of Edinburgh

Allett, N, Keightley, E & Pickering, M (2011) 'Realities toolkit #16: using self-interviews to research memory', *Realities at the Morgan Centre*, Manchester: The University of Manchester

Allmark, P, Boote, J, Chambers, E, Clarke, A, McDonnell, A, Thompson, A & Tod, A M (2009) 'Ethical issues in the use of in-depth interviews: literature review and discussion', *Research Ethics Review*, 5, 48–54

Ameriks, K (2000) 'Introduction', in K Ameriks, Ed., *The Cambridge Companion to German Idealism*, Cambridge: Cambridge University Press, 1–17

Arber, Agnes (1950) *The Natural Philosophy of Plant Form*, Cambridge: Cambridge University Press

Atkinson, Robert (2007) 'The life story interview as a bridge in narrative inquiry', in D J Clandinin, Ed., *Handbook of Narrative Inquiry: Mapping a Methodology*, Thousand Oaks: SAGE Publications, 224–247

Beiser, F (2005) *Schiller as Philosopher: A Re-examination*, Oxford: Oxford University Press

Benn, Sheila (1991) 'Friedrich Schiller and the English Garden: Über den Gartenkalender auf das Jahr 1795', *Garden History*, 19, 1, 28–46

Bentley, Susan M (2009) *Friedrich Schiller's Play: A Theory of Human Nature in the Context of the Eighteenth-century Study of Life*, PhD thesis, Louisville: University of Louisville

Bernstein, J M (2002) *Classic and Romantic German Aesthetics*, Cambridge: Cambridge University Press

Bingley, A F, McDermott, E, Thomas, C, Payne, S (2006) 'Making sense of dying: a review of narratives written since 1950 by people facing death from cancer and other diseases', *Palliative Medicine*, 20, 183–195

Bishop, Paul (2005) 'Reaction and Revolution in Thomas Mann', *Oxford German Studies*, 34, 158–172

Bishop, Paul (2015) 'Goethe and morphology', *Metascience*, 24, 81–83

Bornat, J (2008) 'Biographical Methods', in P Alasuutari, L Bickman, & J Brannen, Eds, *The SAGE Handbook of Social Research Methods*, London: SAGE Publications, 344–356

Bortoft, Henri (1996) *The Wholeness of Nature: Goethe's Way of Science*, Edinburgh: Floris Books

Boufoy-Bastick, Béatrice (2004) 'Auto-interviewing, auto-ethnography and critical incident methodology for eliciting a self-conceptualised worldview', *Forum: Qualitative Social Research*, 5, 1, 1–14

Brown, Jane K (2009) 'Romanticism and Classicism', in N Saul, *The Cambridge Companion to German Romanticism*, Cambridge: Cambridge University Press, 119–132

Bruner, E M (1986) 'Ethnography as narrative', in V Turner & E M Bruner, Eds, *The Anthropology of Experience*, Urbana: University of Illinois Press

Butler-Kisber, Lynn (2010) *Qualitative Inquiry: Thematic, Narrative and Arts-informed Perspectives*, London: SAGE

Byatt, A S (2005) 'Introduction', in Thomas Mann, *The Magic Mountain*, London: Everyman's Library

Campion-Smith, Charles, Austin, Helen, Criswick, Sue, Dowling, Beryl, & Francis, Graham (2011) 'Can sharing stories change practice? A qualitative study of an interprofessional narrative-based palliative care course', *Journal of Interprofessional Care*, 25, 105–111

Capra, Fritjof (1975) *The Tao of Physics*, Boulder: Shambala

Chandler, D (2002) *Semiotics: The Basics*, Hove: Psychology Press

Charon, Rita (2006) *Narrative Medicine: Honoring the Stories of Illness*, Oxford: Oxford University Press

Clandinin, D J & Connelly, F M (2000) *Narrative Inquiry: Experience and Story in Qualitative Research*, San Francisco: Jossey-Bass Publishers

Clandinin, D J & Huber, J (2010) 'Narrative inquiry', in J Huber, B McGaw, E Baker & P Peterson, Eds, *International Encyclopedia of Education*, New York: Elsevier, 436–441

Clandinin, D J & Rosiek, J (2007) 'Mapping a landscape of narrative inquiry: borderland spaces and tensions', in D J Clandinin, Ed., *Handbook of Narrative Inquiry: Mapping a Methodology*, Thousand Oaks: SAGE Publications, 35–77

Clow, B (2001) 'Who's afraid of Susan Sontag? Or, the myths and metaphors of cancer reconsidered', *Social History of Medicine*, 14, 2, 293–312

Coates, Kimberly Engdahl (2012) 'Phantoms, fancy (and) symptoms: Virginia Woolf and the art of being ill', *Woolf Studies Annual*, 18, 1–28

Connelly, F Michael & Clandinin, D Jean (1990) 'Stories of experience and narrative inquiry', *Educational Researcher*, 19, 5, 2–14

Craib, Ian (2003) 'Fear, death and sociology', *Mortality*, 8, 3, 285–295

Craig, Charlotte M (2005) 'Schiller's relevance for us and for all times: a tribute to Friedrich Schiller to commemorate the 200th anniversary of his death', *Logos*, 4, 2

Cristiano, G (2008) *The Storyboard Design Course: The Ultimate Guide for Artists, Directors, Producers and Scriptwriters*, London: Thames & Hudson

Croxton, Derek (1999) 'The peace of Westphalia of 1648 and the origins of sovereignty', *The International History Review*, 21, 569–591

Dahlstrom, Daniel (2000) 'The aesthetic holism of Hamann, Herder and Schiller', in K Ameriks, Ed., *The Cambridge Companion to German Idealism*, Cambridge: Cambridge University Press

Dahlstrom, Daniel O (2011) 'Play and irony: Schiller and Schlegel on the liberating prospects of aesthetics', in T Nenon, Ed., *Kant, Kantianism, and Idealism*, Chicago: University of Chicago Press, 107–129

Ellis, Carolyn (1993) '"There are survivors": telling a story of sudden death', *The Sociological Quarterly*, 34, 4, 711–730

Ellis, Carolyn (2007) 'Telling secrets, revealing lives: relational ethics in research with intimate others', *Qualitative Inquiry*, 13, 1, 3–29

Ellis, C, Adams, T E, & Bochner, A P (2011) 'Autoethnography: an overview', *Historical Social Research*, 36, 4, 273–290

Ellis, C & Bochner, A P (2000) 'Authoethnography, personal narrative, reflexivity: researcher as subject', in N K Denzin & Y S Lincoln, Eds, *Handbook of Qualitative Research*, Thousand Oaks: SAGE, 733–768

Fawcett, Tonks N (2011) 'Cancer: a journey of discovery', in J Fawcett & A McQueen, Eds, *Perspectives on Cancer Care*, Oxford: Blackwell Publishing Ltd

Finnegan, R (1992) *Oral Traditions and the Verbal Arts: A Guide to Research Practices*, London: Routledge

Frank, Arthur W (2000) 'The standpoint of storyteller', *Qualitative Health Research*, 10, 354–365

Frank, Arthur W (2010) *Letting Stories Breathe: A Socio-narratology*, Chicago: University of Chicago Press

Frankenberg, R (1988) '"Your time or mine". An anthropological view of the tragic temporal contradictions of biomedical practice', *International Journal of Health Services*, 1, 11–34

Freedman, D, Thornton, A, Camburn, D, Alwin, D & Young-Demarco, L (1988) 'The life history calendar: a technique for collecting retrospective data', *Sociological Methodology*, 18, 37–68

Froggatt, K A (1995) *Keeping the Balance: Hospice Work, Death and Emotions*, PhD thesis, South Bank University

Froggatt, K (1997) 'Rites of passage and the hospice culture', *Mortality*, 2, 123–136

Froggatt, K (1998) 'The place of metaphor and language in exploring nurses' emotional work', *Journal of Advanced Nursing*, 28, 2, 332–338

Galvin, Kathleen & Todres, Les (2007) 'The creativity of "unspecialization": a contemplative direction for integrative scholarly practice', *Phenomenology & Practice*, 1, 31–46

Galvin, Kathleen T & Todres, Les (2011) 'Research based empathic knowledge for nursing: a translational strategy for disseminating phenomenological research findings to provide evidence for caring practice', *International Journal of Nursing Studies*, 48, 4, 522–530

Geertz, C (1973) 'Thick description: toward an interpretive theory of culture', in *The Interpretation of Culture: Selected Essays*, New York: Basic Books, 3–30.

Gendlin, E T (2004) 'The new phenomenology of carrying forward', *Continental Philosophy Review*, 37, 1, 127–151

George, Linda K (2002) 'Research design in end-of-life research: state of science', *The Gerontologist*, 42, 86–98

Gesler, Wil (2000) 'Hans Castorp's journey-to-knowledge of disease and health in Thomas Mann's *The Magic Mountain*', *Health & Place*, 6, 2, 125–134

Goethe, Johann Wolfgang (1906) *Maxims and Reflections*, New York: The Macmillan Company

Goethe, Johann Wolfgang (1970) *Theory of Colours*, Cambridge: MIT Press

Goethe, Johann Wolfgang (2016) *The Essential Goethe*, Princeton: Princeton University Press

Greenberg, Valerie D (1985) 'Literature and the discourse of science: the paradigm of Thomas Mann's "The Magic Mountain"', *South Atlantic Review*, 50, 1, 59–73

Grossmann, Walter (1968) 'Schiller's Aesthetic Education', *Journal of Aesthetic Education*, 2, 31–41

Hammermeister, K (2002) *The German Aesthetic Tradition*, Cambridge: Cambridge University Press

Hawkins, Anne H (1993) *Reconstructing Illness: Studies in Pathography*, West Lafayette: Purdue University Press

Heilferty, C M (2009) 'Toward a theory of online communication in illness: concept analysis of illness blogs', *Journal of Advanced Nursing*, 65, 7, 1539–1547
Heinemann, Fritz (1934) 'Goethe's phenomenological method', *Philosophy*, 9, 33, 67–81
Holdrege, Craig (2005) 'Doing Goethean science', *Janus Head*, 8, 1, 27–52
Hunt, Celia (2013) *Transformative Learning through Creative Life Writing: Exploring the Self in the Learning Process*, London: Routledge
Jack, B & O'Brien, M (2010) 'Dying at home: community nurses' views on the impact of informal carers on cancer patients' place of death', *European Journal of Cancer Care*, 19, 5, 636–642
Jacobs, Don (Four Arrows) (2008) *The Authentic Dissertation*, Abingdon: Routledge
Janesick, V M (1998) 'The dance of qualitative research design: metaphor, methodolatry, and meaning', in N K Denzin, & Y S Lincoln, Eds, *Handbook of Qualitative Research*, Thousand Oaks: SAGE, 209–219
Jarvis, Peter (1995) *Adult and Continuing Education: Theory and Practice*, London: Routledge
Jones, Kip (2003) 'The turn to a narrative knowing of persons: one method explored', *Journal of Research in Nursing*, 8, 1, 60–71
Kellehear, Allan (2014) *The Inner Life of the Dying Person*, New York: Columbia University Press
Kendall, M, Murray, S A, Carduff, E, Worth, A, Harris, F, Lloyd, A, Cavers, D, Sheikh, A (2010) 'Use of multiperspective qualitative interviews to understand patients' and carers' beliefs, experiences, and needs', *British Medical Journal*, 340
Kennedy, John F (1961) *President Kennedy's Inaugural Address*
Kim, S (2009) 'Content analysis of cancer blog posts', *Journal of the Medical Library Association*, 97, 4, 260–266
Kimball, Roger (2001) 'Schiller's "Aesthetic Education"', *New Criterion*, 19, 12–19
Knowles, J G & Promislow, S (2008) 'Using an arts methodology to create a thesis or dissertation', in J G Knowles & A L Cole, Eds, *Handbook of the Arts in Qualitative Research: Perspectives, Methodologies, Examples, and Issues*, Thousand Oaks: SAGE Publications, 511–527
Kvale, S (2007) *Doing Interviews*, London: SAGE Publications Ltd
Lakoff, G & Johnson, M (1980) 'Conceptual metaphor in everyday language', *The Journal of Philosophy*, 77, 8, 453–486
Lambek, M (2003) 'Introduction: irony and illness – recognition and refusal', *Social Analysis*, 47, 2, 1–19
Langellier, K M (1999) 'Personal narrative, performance, performativity: two or three things I know for sure', *Text and Performance Quarterly*, 19, 125–144
Langellier, K M (2003) 'Personal narrative, performance, performativity: two or three things I know for sure', in Yvonne S Lincoln, & Norman K Denzin, Eds, *Turning Points in Qualitative Research: Tying Knots in the Handkerchief*, Walnut Creek: AltaMira Press
Lawton, Julia (1998) 'Contemporary hospice care: the sequestration of the unbounded body and "dirty dying"', *Sociology of Health & Illness*, 20, 2, 121–143
MacLaren, Jessica (2014) *Making Sense of Supervision: A Narrative Study of the Supervision Experiences of Mental Health Nurses and Midwives*, PhD thesis, Edinburgh: University of Edinburgh.
Mahoney, D (2002) 'Autobiographical writings', in L Sharpe, Ed., *The Cambridge Companion to Goethe*, Cambridge: Cambridge University Press, 147–159
Mann, Thomas (2005) *The Magic Mountain*, London: Everyman's Library
Márquez, Gabriel García (1988) *Love in the Time of Cholera*, London: Jonathan Cape Ltd
McGilchrist, Iain (2012) *The Master and his Emissary: The Divided Brain and the Making of the Western World*, New Haven, CT: Yale University Press
Nehamas, A (1998) *The Art of Living: Socratic Reflections from Plato to Foucault*, Berkley: University of California Press

Nordgren, S & Fridlund, B (2001) 'Patients' perceptions of self-determination as expressed in the context of care', *Journal of Advanced Nursing*, 35, 117–125

O'Brien, Mary R & Clark, David (2010) 'Use of unsolicited first-person written illness narratives in research: systematic review', *Journal of Advanced Nursing*, 66, 1671–1682

Oosterwijk, S & Knöll, S A (2011) *Mixed Metaphors: The Danse Macabre in Medieval and Early Modern Europe*, Newcastle upon Tyne: Cambridge Scholars

Open Book (2013) 'Bernard MacLaverty on a literary life', *Open Book*, London: BBC Radio 4

Payne, S (2010) 'White Paper on improving support for family carers in palliative care', *European Journal of Palliative Care*, 17, 5, 238–290

Pierret, J (2003) 'The illness experience: state of knowledge and perspectives for research', *Sociology of Health & Illness*, 25, 3, 4–22

Plenderleith, Helen Jane (1991) *The Testament of Dichtung und Wahrheit: An Enquiry into Goethe's Mode of Secularization*, PhD thesis, Glasgow: University of Glasgow

Plenderleith, Helen Jane (1993) 'An approach to Goethe's treatment of religion in Dichtung und Wahrheit', *German Life and Letters*, 46, 297–310

Plummer, K (2001) *Documents of Life 2: An Invitation to a Critical Humanism*, London: SAGE

Redding, Paul (2011) 'German Idealism', in G Klosko, *The Oxford Handbook of the History of Political Philosophy*, Oxford: Oxford University Press

Reed, T J (2002) 'Weimar classicism: Goethe's alliance with Schiller', in Lesley Sharpe, Ed., *The Cambridge Companion to Goethe*, Cambridge: University of Cambridge Press, 101–115

Richards, Robert J (2002) *The Romantic Conception of Life: Science and Philosophy in the Age of Goethe*, Chicago: University of Chicago Press

Richardson, L (2000) 'Writing: a method of inquiry', in N K Denzin, & Y S Lincoln, Eds, *Handbook of Qualitative Research*, Thousand Oaks: SAGE, 923–948

Riessman, C K (2004) 'A thrice-told tale: new readings of an old story', in B Hurwitz, T, Greenhalgh & V Skultans, Eds, *Narrative Research in Health and Illness*, Oxford: Blackwell, 309–324

Riessman, C K (2008) *Narrative Methods for the Human Sciences*, Los Angeles: SAGE Publications

Riessman, C K & Speedy, J (2007) 'Narrative inquiry in the psychotherapy professions: a critical review' in D J Clandinin, Ed., *Handbook of Narrative Inquiry: Mapping a Methodology*, Thousand Oaks: SAGE Publications, 426–457

Rosch, Eleanor (1987) 'Linguistic relativity', *ETC: A Review of General Semantics*, 254–279

Schaper, Eva (1985) 'Towards the aesthetic: a journey with Friedrich Schiller', *The British Journal of Aesthetics*, 25, 2, 153–168

Scheper-Hughes, N & Lock, M M (1986) 'Speaking "truth" to illness: metaphors, reification, and a pedagogy for patients', *Medical Anthropology Quarterly*, 17, 137–140

Schiller, Friedrich (1954) *On the Aesthetic Education of Man in a Series of Letters*, Trans. R Snell, New Haven: Yale University Press

Schiller, Friedrich (2016) *On the Aesthetic Education of Man in a Series of Letters*, Trans. K Tribe, with Notes by A Schmidt, London: Penguin Random House

Schindler, D C (2008) 'An aesthetics of freedom: Friedrich Schiller's breakthrough beyond subjectivism', *Yearbook of the Irish Philosophical Society*, 84–109

Schmitz, L D (1877) *Correspondence between Schiller and Goethe, from 1794 to 1797: Translated from the Third Edition of the German with Notes*, London: George Bell

Schmitz, L D (1890) *Correspondence between Schiller and Goethe, from 1798 to 1805: Translated from the Third Edition of the German with Notes*, London: George Bell

Seamon, David (1998) 'Goethe, nature and phenomenology', in David Seamon & Arthur Zajonc, Eds, *Goethe's Way of Science: A Phenomenology of Nature*, Albany, NY: State University of New York Press

Seamon, David (2005) 'Goethe's way of science as a phenomenology of nature', *Janus Head*, 8, 1, 86–101

Sehn, Zoe L (2013) *Creating Meaning in the Face of Bereavement: An Adult Child's Perspective*, Professional Doctorate in Psychotherapy and Counselling, Edinburgh: University of Edinburgh

Sharp, Henry Stephen (1996) 'Experiencing meaning', *Anthropology and Humanism*, 21, 2, 171–186

Sharpe, Lesley (1991) *Friedrich Schiller: Drama, Thought and Politics*, Cambridge: Cambridge University Press

Sharpe, Lesley (2002) 'Introduction', in Lesley Sharpe, Ed., *The Cambridge Companion to Goethe*, Cambridge: Cambridge University Press, 1–5

Shotter, John (2000) 'Seeing historically: Goethe and Vygotsky's "enabling theory-method"', *Culture & Psychology*, 6, 233–252

Skott, C (2002) 'Expressive metaphors in cancer narratives', *Cancer Nursing*, 25, 3, 230–235

SOED (2007) *Shorter Oxford English Dictionary*, Oxford: Oxford University Press

Solzhenitsyn, Aleksandr (1970) *Cancer Ward*, London: The Bodley Head Ltd

Sontag, S (1978) *Illness as Metaphor*, Harmondsworth: Penguin

Squire, C, Andrews, M & Tamboukou, M (2008) 'Introduction: What is narrative research?' in M Andrews, C Squire & M Tamboukou, Eds, *Doing Narrative Research*, London: SAGE Publications, 1–22

Stacey, Jackie (1997) *Teratologies: A Cultural Study of Cancer*, London: Routledge

Stanley, Liz (1992) *The Auto/biographical I: The Theory and Practice of Feminist Auto/biography*, Manchester: Manchester University Press

Stanley, Liz (1993) 'The knowing because experiencing subject: narratives, lives and autobiography', *Women's Studies International Forum*, 16, 3, 205–215

Stanley, Liz (2012) 'Whites writing: letters and documents of life in a QLR project', in Liz Stanley, Ed., *Documents of Life Revisited: Narrative & Biographical Methods for a 21st Century Critical Humanism*, Farnham: Ashgate Publishing, 1–21

Stanley, Liz & Temple, Bogusia (2008) 'Narrative methodologies: subjects, silences, re-readings and analyses', *Qualitative Research*, 8, 275–281

Stephenson, R H (1983) *Goethe's Wisdom Literature: A Study in Aesthetic Transmutation*, Oxford: Peter Lang

Stephenson, R H (1995) *Mind at Work: Goethe's Conception of Knowledge and Science*, Edinburgh: Edinburgh University Press

Stephenson, R H (2005) '"Binary synthesis": Goethe's aesthetic intuition in literature and science', *Science in Context*, 18, 4, 553–581

Steuer, Daniel (2002) 'In defence of experience', in Lesley Sharpe, Ed., *The Cambridge Companion to Goethe*, Cambridge: University of Cambridge Press, 160–178

Swales, M (2002) 'Goethe's prose fiction', in Lesley Sharpe, Ed., *The Cambridge Companion to Goethe*, Cambridge: Cambridge University Press, 129–146

Thomas, C (2009) *Narratives of Living and Dying with Cancer: Sociological Perspectives*, Swindon: ESRC

Todres, Les (2008) 'Being with that: the relevance of embodied understanding for practice', *Qualitative Health Research*, 18, 11, 1566–1573

Todres, Les & Galvin, Kathleen T (2008) 'Embodied interpretation: a novel way of evocatively re-presenting meanings in phenomenological research', *Qualitative Research*, 8, 5, 568–583

van Manen, Max (2006) 'Writing qualitatively, or the demands of writing', *Qualitative Health Research*, 16, 5, 713–722

van Manen, Max (2007) 'Phenomenology of practice', *Phenomenology & Practice*, 1, 11–30

van Manen, Max (2014) *Phenomenology of Practice*, Walnut Creek: Left Coast Press
Voltaire (2008) *Candide and Other Stories*, Oxford World's Classics, Oxford: Oxford University Press
Wahl, Daniel C (2005) '"Zarte Empirie": Goethean science as a way of knowing', *Janus Head*, 8, 1, 58–76
Wengraf, Tom (2000) 'Uncovering the general from the particular', in P Chamberlayne, J Bornat & T Wengraf, Eds, *The Turn to Biographical Methods in Social Science*, London: Routledge
Wilkinson, E M (1948) 'Goethe's botany by Agnes Arber', *The Modern Language Review*, 43, 556–558
Wilkinson, E M (1955) 'Schiller's concept of Schein in the light of recent aesthetics', *The German Quarterly*, 28, 219–227
Wilkinson, E M (1959) '"Form" and "content" in the aesthetics of German Classicism', in P Böckmann, Ed., *Stil- und Formprobleme in der Literatur*, Vorträge des VII Kongresses der Internationalen Vereinigung für Moderne Sprachen und Literaturen in Heidelberg, Heidelberg: Carl Winter, 18–27
Wilkinson, E M & Willoughby, L A (1962) *Goethe: Poet and Thinker*, London: Hodder & Stoughton
Wilkinson, E M & Willoughby, L A (1967) *On the Aesthetic Education of Man in a Series of Letters*, Oxford: Clarendon Press
Wilkinson, E M & Willoughby, L A (2002) '"The Whole Man" in Schiller's theory of culture and society', in J D Adler, M Swales, & A C Weaver, Eds, *Models of Wholeness: Some Attitudes to Language, Art and Life in the Age of Goethe*, Oxford: Peter Lang
Williams, John R (1998) *The Life of Goethe: A Critical Biography*, Wiley-Blackwell: Oxford
Woolf, Virginia (2012) *On Being Ill: With Notes from Sick Rooms by Julia Stephen*, Ashfield MA: Paris Press
Yao C, Hu W, Lai Y, Cheng S, Chen C Y & Chiu T Y (2007) 'Does dying at home influence the good death of terminal cancer patients?', *Journal of Pain and Symptom Management*, 34, 5, 497–504
Zajonc, A (1998) 'Goethe and the phenomenological investigation of consciousness', in S Hammeroff, A Kaszniak & D Chalmers, Eds, *Toward a Science of Consciousness III*, Cambridge: MIT Press

2
INVITATION TO THE DANCE

Having struggled with the *best* way to present the data and after many iterations, I arrived at an approach similar to that previously described as *embodied relational understanding* (Todres, 2008). This chapter and the next two report the Illness Period, the time from when Jane became unwell to when she died, as *The Dance to Death*. In this writing I have attempted a style of expression where "embodied interpretation is [used] to communicate findings in more evocative ways that may support readers in understanding, in an empathic way, what a phenomenon may be like" (Todres & Galvin, 2008: 580). The process can be considered a *return enhanced* to the witness testimony of my experience now re-appreciated through understanding from the academic literature. This could also be expressed as an interaction between *heart* as experience and *head* as objective truth as enacted by the *hand* of the research process.

Ethical considerations are addressed by anonymising references to others and using their relationship or role in square brackets: [my sister], [the surgeon]. The analytic narrative as an embodied appreciation of the shared illness experience begins just before Jane's diagnosis and is told in three chapters that reflect the three phases of the Illness Period which as a whole are *The Dance to Death*. Each chapter has three episodes with titles that reflect the defining themes for the phase. There are no subsections within the episodes to avoid interrupting the narrative flow. The first chapter details events from the first two months of the Illness Period with the episodes: Wondering, Finding, and Planning. At approximately six weeks this is the shortest period addressed in the chapters.

Some background to *The Dance to Death* is needed before the actual illness narrative begins. After ten hectic years of running our own educational consultancy we had grown weary with the effort and decided to embark on a new adventure. Our plan was for a quieter life in north-eastern France, nearer to our mutual interests of food, wine, walking and cycling. Getting there was a huge undertaking that left us both exhausted, drained and trying to survive the winter in a small caravan (Lotte) with two grumpy cats and temperatures of −20°C. After a month of cold angst, we abandoned the plan and made our way slowly back to Scotland. We stayed with my brother in Belgium to pass the two months required by quarantine regulations before our cats could re-enter the UK. As we had no permanent home, we headed for Glasgow and temporary lodgings with Jane's mother. We could have chosen to live anywhere in Scotland but decided on a flat in Edinburgh with a decent garden and a view of the nearby Pentland hills. During this time Jane had kept a blog to keep family and friends informed of our adventures but it was outwith the timeframe for the original study. However, there are some posts, all written by Jane, which perhaps give a more accurate impression of her than my personal and inevitably very biased recollections. So a brief interlude for some relevant blog episodes from just before the story proper, anonymised but with place names and dates retained.

Prequel

> Yesterday afternoon I got my finger caught in the caravan door. This being a rather well-built caravan with a sturdy frame, and the door having been closed with some force, the injury is not trivial. [Veronica] realised this immediately and wheeched me off to the nearest A & E. My first personal visit to casualty in at least 20 years and things do seem to have changed. Not least a fixation with waiting time targets (no more than 4 hours) and a tremendous generosity with the use of dressings. Two very nice nurse practitioners pronounced the injury beyond them, and having prescribed antibiotics and painkillers sent me off to see a plastics specialist in Slough (come, friendly bombs…).
>
> Said specialist pronounced the injury to be 'spectacular' and one of the most interesting referrals he's had in a while. So I'm a teaching case as well as a basket case. There's an open fracture, (a Type 2 Mallet finger), crush injury, tendon damage, and possible nerve damage. We've to go back to Slough tomorrow morning for a wee operation, under local anaesthetic, which will hopefully save the shape and functionality of my left index finger. I suspect that's the end to any chance of a late career change to concert pianist, guitarist or hand model. But hopefully I'll be able to type using both hands again in a couple of months.
>
> I'll be in a stookie for a few days (actually I'm not sure the young man who saw me today knew what a stookie is) and then have to go back to have a custom splint made. That and the continuing bad weather are conspiring to keep us in England. We are having to be patient in a number of senses.
>
> *(Blog post, 'Accident & Emergency', 1 December 2010)*

> It's been an odd week at Chertsey. We've not been able to move out of this little corner west of London on account of the weather which seems to have

paralysed most of the rest of the country, blocked the channel tunnel and caused problems in northern France too.

We spent most of Thursday in the waiting room of the Day Surgery unit in Slough. Turned up as requested shortly after 8, and I was eventually taken to theatre at half past three. Was treated by a very nice young registrar who seemed quite dismissive at first ('we'll just splint your fingers together and you'll always have some stiffness') but changed her mind when I explained what I would like to happen in terms of maximising functionality and minimising deformity (thanks to [Veronica's] research into Type 2 Mallet fingers) and she saw the wound. Her anticipated ten-minute rush job turned into a meticulous 45-minute repair. I've got internal and external stitching including a nail bed laceration repair and an internal wire (with a hook at the end, so beware ticking crocodiles). And I got to see the inside of an operating theatre for the first time, which was fascinating. Under local anaesthetic so I could hear what was being said and chat to the surgeons (how ER is that?) but no mirrors and they wouldn't let me watch.

Then yesterday morning we went back to the hand clinic where the nice young SHO (there is a pattern developing here) whom we saw on Wednesday morning wrote a detailed 'To whom it may concern' letter for me to take to a specialist somewhere else (eg France) explaining the treatment I've received and suggesting the aftercare regime that's required in order to remove the wire. Then I had the wound redressed (under [Veronica's] supervision) and went to Rehab (saying no, no, no) to have a custom splint fitted. All sorted by lunchtime and we were free to go.

I've had more dealings with the NHS over the last four days than I've had in at least forty years. I've always thought of myself as a net contributor rather than beneficiary of the NHS. I've been really touched by the kindness, care and professionalism of all the staff I've come into contact with – from the A & E nurse practitioners, the specialist hand clinic, day surgery unit, theatre staff and rehab clinic [in Slough]. However, I've been less than impressed with the NHS systems and management practices. It took almost 48 hours from injury to repair which is ok but not great, not least because I spent eight hours unnecessarily waiting around with an open fracture risking infection. We had to make four return trips to two different hospitals, a cumulative distance of about 120 miles. We paid quite a lot of money for hospital car parking. There wasn't anything worth eating (with any nutritional value) available in the hospital canteen. The nurses seemed to have to spend a lot of time and effort filling in forms (I had the distinct impression that the nurse who did my post-op checks was more concerned with ticking the box that said she'd taken my blood pressure than actually reviewing what the reading might mean in terms of my health).

But all is well, my left index finger is safe in its little plastic cradle, [Veronica] has made me a lovely mitten so I can still do the washing up and fetch the water, and two days after the op I am no longer demanding painkillers at minimum intervals. We leave for France this week.

(Blog post, 'Sorted', 4 December 2010)

We've been thinking and talking a lot over the past few days about the notion of 'home' and what it means. Home for the last six weeks or so has been Lotte, wherever she is, a little hermetically sealed bubble where we are warm and comfortable and safe, with our things and of course our cats. But at an even more fundamental level home is a geographical concept, a place with which we identify, for whatever reasons. For me, it's quite clear that home is Glasgow because that's where I know myself to be from, and where almost everyone with whom I have a blood relation still lives. For [Veronica] that's a bit less clear since she left the place where she brought up when she was eighteen, and her immediate family is scattered across several countries in two continents. But her chosen home from the age of eighteen was Edinburgh, so in that sense both of us are at home in Scotland.

Home is where the heart is. That's easy then, physiologically speaking at least, home is where I am physically present, as long as I have a pulse. But emotionally inexplicable – is one's heart with a person, a place, a set of circumstances? Wherever I lay my hat, that's my home. What's the cultural and emotional charge in the notion of laying one's hat? Maybe it's easier to understand what is not home. Home is not here. Here is not home. Here feels quite strange, even when we enjoy and appreciate the strangeness, it's still strange. In German, home is 'Heim'. But 'heimlich' (literally 'homely') means secret, kept to oneself, not shared. And 'unheimlich' means weird, uncanny, unnatural. Not being at home means being uneasy. One thing at least is clear – home is not and will not be Alsace. Lovely as it is, we will not be making a home for ourselves here. We'll be taking our little portable home somewhere else where we feel more at ease.

(Blog post, 'Home', 27 December 2010)

It's been five weeks since the accident and operation, so it was time for the wire to come out. Sister Adamson performed the procedure successfully yesterday morning (and I wasn't allowed to look). [My brother] the sometime orthopaedic technician has fashioned me a replacement splint from a bit of reclaimed aluminium and some velcro. We're not sure whether to paint a knight's face (I call it Roland) or make some snail antennae ([my brother] calls it Brian). At any rate it's a relief no longer to be wired up and have a bit more movement in the finger. Also to have achieved all stages of the post-op care so far without needing to use the medic-to-medic letter they gave me in the hospital in Slough which started 'Thank you for seeing this 50-year-old woman…' because I felt that was an unnecessary detail. I'm keeping the pin as a souvenir – my Grandma Plenderleith would have had it for a hat-pin :)

(Blog post, 'Finger Update', 7 January 2011)

We had epiphany cake (*galette des rois, driekoningentaart*) today, brought from a market in Brussels this morning. And I got the bean. I confess I didn't know what epiphany cake was until a couple of days ago. A quick Google search indicates that there are lots of variations on this theme in many different countries. There's some kind of trinket inside each cake and the person who gets it in their slice gets to wear a crown and be king or queen for the year. The trinket is called *une fève* here, so presumably it was indeed originally some kind of dried bean. My bean is a little porcelain drummer boy (that's appropriate in this house). The cake, by the way, is a kind of almond pithivier in a delicious flaky butter pastry. I heard before we left France that a baker in the south had put real gold coins in some of his galettes des rois so there was a bit of a run on his cakes.

(Blog post, 'Epiphany', 9 January 2011)

So here we are back in Scotland, in the middle of March, and it's still snowing. If I haven't blogged much about our impending return, that's because we were quite busy with things to do in Belgium before we went, and packing and planning for another grand départ, this time in the opposite direction.

It's funny how things turn out. From Belgium we knew we could hitch our caravan to the back of the car and head off for far-flung places (I often cited Vladivostok as a theoretical possibility, but had no real answer to [Veronica's] 'why on earth would you want to go there?') but really where we think we want to be is [here].

Quite a lot of taxpayers' money (and my parents' hard-won resources) was invested in my education over several decades. It will come as no surprise to many and perhaps small relief to some that some ideas, concepts, maxims, tropes and truisms from eighteenth century German literature and philosophy continue to colour my (our) thinking today. [Veronica] and I have often made reference to binary synthesis, a synthesis of polarised opposites, in our work and even with reference to ourselves. And what we are now experiencing is very much a return enhanced.

We've towed our caravan all the way through England and quite a lot of France and Belgium. We've learned to live small (it's surprising how few tools, books, clothes and various accoutrements are actually essential). We've lived in a community with many different people, doing weird and wonderful things. We've shopped and cooked and cleaned in many different circumstances of varying comfort. We've experienced different cultures and traditions. We've kept it together through some quite challenging and difficult times and have emerged stronger and more sure of what matters in life.

We've written reports, held meetings and discussions, organised various initiatives and kept in touch with key contacts and secured more work contracts while we've been away. The cats have been through a lot with us and have been quite stoical throughout. They've learned to tolerate one another, and take changing circumstances in their stride. They hate moving, especially in the car (they managed the ferry no bother) but cope with living in different places and spaces. Curiously they are showing very little interest in the outside world, wherever they are.

> Tea has never tasted better. We may bemoan the weather, but the seemingly constant precipitation in various levels of solidity which falls on the rocks of Scotland does produce wonderfully soft water for which we have a renewed appreciation. Likewise the wind you can really fill your lungs with and breathe deeply again.
>
> It's special to be back among our family and friends here. Some of them have actually held onto much of the stuff we gave away before we left, because they knew we'd be back. Many years ago [Veronica] chose to come and live in Scotland. I never did – it was simply home, where I lived, no question, point final. Now, having been where we've been and seen what we've seen, we have chosen to come back. Truly a return enhanced.
>
> *(Blog post, 'Return Enhanced', 15 March 2011)*

Wondering

This first story of *The Dance to Death* begins two months before realising something was wrong. During this time Jane becomes unwell, shortly after our return from a visit to London. A month is spent visiting GPs (general practitioners) as we attempt to discover the cause of her unwell feelings while also purchasing our flat in Edinburgh. The first suggestion that Jane is not feeling as fit as she once had, comes in a blog posting where she reflects on a day's hill walking on Ben Lomond:

> The views were splendid, if a little hazy, and I had a grand time to myself recognising old friends. The Cobbler and the rest of the Arrochar Alps, Ben More and Stob Binnein, Ben Lawers and 'that wee pointy bastard in the distance' which, as Muriel Gray memorably remarked, is always Schiehallion. There were cows and calves grazing near the path, butterworts, harebells and violets bright flashes of colour along the way, and the loch shining deep and blue below Ptarmigan ridge.
>
> I thought I was fine in my new boots, striding up the path, sure-footed on the slight scrambly bits off the top, but boy did I suffer later. Thigh muscles so sore and tight that each normal walking step was painful for several days afterwards. So a few lessons learned. Mountain climbing in your 50s is not the same as mountain climbing in your 20s. The days of bouncing up and back down again in three hours or so are long gone.
>
> *(Blog post, 'Ben Lomond', 5 June 2011)*

To me this illustrates the essential Jane, someone who loved and knew the Scottish mountains, full of energy and enthusiasm for adventure yet innocently bemused by her apparently recalcitrant body. It also demonstrates her aesthetic appreciation of the scenery in terms of both the macro grandeur and the micro detail of particular wild flowers. I recall the walk in my first interview and the curious difference in our fitness.

Well, throughout the time we'd been travelling about we'd done various things to kind of maintain a level of fitness so we'd gone for walks every day but in the winter you know it was −20 and deep snow but nevertheless we did go out every day. It was extremely difficult to do yoga in a very small caravan so I had a kind of variation where we would go over to the shower block and do some sort of yoga. And then when we were staying with her mum, Jane increasingly had this low back pain. I believed [it] was to do with tension and stress and that we could fix it by doing more exercises. But the hill walking, Jane was younger than me and had always been ahead on the hill, faster than me, more fearless, more gallous. But we seemed to be much more evenly matched and I really noticed that she did complain for days afterwards about how sore her legs were.

And then I think it was either one or two weeks later we did this long walk which was a bit easier going and it was a lovely walk but she didn't have the pace that she had previously. But I didn't particularly notice that at the time, we were just enjoying the walk and pleased to have made the decision to be in Scotland and to have found the flat.

(Interview One, 9 July 2013)

These vague symptoms of low back pain and fatigue are typical of ovarian cancer, the 'silent killer' (McCorkle et al., 2003) that creeps insidiously hidden deep within its unsuspecting host. In this excerpt is probably the essence of me as partner – pragmatic, caring, philosophical and with the overwhelming sense of accountability characteristic of the eldest child: if something has gone wrong, it is your responsibility and you must try to fix it (preferably prior to discovery). While I recognise and accept that I was in no way responsible for Jane's illness, I now wonder if there were two contrasting processes at work. The first is Gadamar's concept of a fusion of horizons and the second is the idea of a mutual conspiracy of silence (Zerubavel, 2006). Gadamer recognised that understanding in the present can only be achieved by acknowledging the prejudices of the past through a "fusion of horizons" (Gadamer, 2004: 306). However, it is not simply the sense of a historical awareness of the past that matters. It is also coming to an understanding through the interpretation placed on a text through our own use of language as a process of questioning and answering (Gadamer, 2004). In the present of recalling in the interview above but now in the past, I was remembering a time many years before when as a nurse I had cared for women with advanced gynaecological cancer. But at the time of the Ben Lomond walk, it was only a vague feeling of uneasiness.

What then of a conspiracy of silence? If I had that awareness, an insight into a serious illness for my partner, why did I remain silent? Furthermore, when Jane observes "the days of bouncing up and back down again in three hours or so are long gone" why does she not question her poor fitness in an apparently otherwise healthy and health-conscious woman in her early fifties? I suggest that we were both mutually yet independently, engaged in a tacit conspiracy of silence.

Zerubavel (2006) reviews the many forms and causes a conspiracy of silence may take, and observes:

> Silent bystanders act as enablers because watching others ignore something encourages one to deny its presence … The discrepancy between others' apparent inability to notice it and one's own sensory experience creates a sense of ambiguity that further increases the likelihood that one would ultimately succumb to the social pressure and opt for denial.
>
> (Zerubavel, 2006: 55)

In the excerpt from my interview, I comment that "I didn't particularly notice that at the time" which seems to confirm Zerubavel's observation. There was a vague change in Jane's stamina, she had noticed her loss of fitness but neither of us voiced any concerns. Pressed by the interviewer on the point of either of us noticing anything to suggest a health issue for Jane, I recall a time some months earlier:

> In Belgium, she said she felt as though she had this brick in her. Because we were displaced, we didn't have a GP [and] we had the language complication despite her fluency and the support that we would have had from the family we were staying with. I think she suspected there was something wrong but she didn't want to be ill in Belgium. She didn't want to be somewhere foreign and be ill.
>
> (Interview One, 9 July 2013)

Despite these indeterminate concerns, we continue with the flat purchase; we also have consultancy work which takes us to London. We travel the day before, stay in our preferred hotel and dine in a favourite restaurant. The following day we return by train; Jane has not been feeling well as I describe:

> This particular evening we'd gone for an Indian meal and I remember being back in the hotel and her abdomen did seem to be distended and she was complaining of bellyache. We had some kind of homoeopathic digestive remedy which she was taking which was helping a bit. Then the following day when we were coming back on the train we had this sort of ritual were we would go and get a picnic so we could have a little evening of the journey, she wasn't feeling particularly hungry, there's a moment, which I remember very, very clearly. When the train had pulled in to Glasgow Central and we're waiting for the doors to unlock, I looked at her and saw this huge distension of her abdomen and very consciously thought 'that looks like ascites but it can't possibly be, that's ridiculous'. I said something to her like 'gosh your belly's really swollen' and she just said 'yes' and she would be glad to get home.
>
> (Interview One, 9 July 2013)

With the still clear memory of her lying on the bed in the hotel in obvious pain and with a very distended abdomen, it seems astonishing that neither of us sought help. It is perhaps understandable that Jane, who again found herself in a foreign land, as England was to her, wanted to wait until she was home, but I had the experience, the knowledge that this could be something very serious. We were very near to a major London teaching hospital but there is no suggestion of doing anything other than trying our own various self-help remedies. There is a clear fusion between my awareness in the then present horizon when the thought arises 'that looks like ascites' and the past horizons of my nursing experience. My thoughts at the time even make use of technical terms that reference medical language. Yet I appear paralysed by our mutual tacit conspiracy that renders us blind to the situation. My memory of the ascites thought remained so clear it became the first day in what I term the Illness Period. My diary entry the following day is a curious mix of clinical observations, therapeutic intervention and witless humour "Jane not feeling that great today – sore back and bellyache. Condition worsened this afternoon and evening – nausea etc, grey, abdomen very distended. Lunch and tea solo!" (Personal diary, 16 June 2011).

The crisis comes during the night when Jane wakes me at 4.30am distressed and crying with the pain but we are not yet registered with a GP. I call the NHS out of hours service and explain the situation and we are instructed to make our way to a nearby treatment centre. Jane is seen promptly by a woman GP who thinks she may have an abdominal obstruction and refers her to the hospital conveniently across the road. I help her to dress and we walk across for her to get undressed again and lie on another hospital trolley. A tall woman comes, the surgical SHO (senior house officer), who examines her and arranges blood tests and x-rays. We wait for about two hours during which time the duty doctors change shifts. The surgical SHO is now a young male doctor. He is cheery and upbeat: apparently constipation and a urinary tract infection (UTI). I am overwhelmed with relief and disbelief, while Jane is:

> just relieved that somebody had given her feeling of unwellness a label. The early hours of that morning she just felt so ill, and then she'd been poked and prodded and x-rayed and all the rest of it and eventually they had pronounced. I was beside myself with worry, I was absolutely convinced there was something very seriously wrong and I remember standing beside her on a trolley in a corridor and just this surge of relief and saying to her 'that's great, that's easily fixed' and her being relieved. But what we didn't understand was why they thought she was constipated, that didn't make sense. She didn't think she was constipated, she'd been constipated before and she knew what that was and she really didn't think she was but they said she was so they supposedly knew better.
>
> *(Interview One, 9 July 2013)*

Antibiotics and a bulking agent are prescribed and we drive home. For the next ten days we persevere with the treatment regime.

She looked very small and pale, with this big tummy, weak, and I had this kind of desperate feeling of wanting her to get better but alongside the antibiotic they'd given her this bulking agent. It was one of those filthy mixtures that you mix up with water and you have to swallow it and she was never very good at swallowing things like that anyway so it was a kind of double whammy, an added punishment. Not only did she feel completely blown up but she had to take this stuff that just seemed to blow her up even more. I kept looking for stuff on the internet about why did she have this abdominal swelling and I was getting answers like a swollen abdomen's ascites and you know why you get ascites [either some sort of malignancy or liver disease]. I kept pushing that away and we kept trying with being obedient and following the treatment that had been prescribed.

(Interview One, 9 July 2013)

The reference to being obedient was because I knew that Jane did not want any fuss made or anything else to draw attention to her condition. But it was perhaps also to maintain the conspiracy of silence – if our unvoiced fears were not acknowledged then this was nothing more than the simple diagnosis that had been made. There were also other events requiring our attention "The flat is now officially ours! It feels right but both somewhat distracted by Jane's enormous belly – think a visit to the new surgery may be in order" (Personal diary, 26 June 2011).

By now Jane's mobility is restricted by what appears to be a full pregnancy, her clothes no longer fit and she spends most nights pacing up and down in considerable discomfort. I register us both with a GP practice near our new home in Edinburgh and she has an appointment on day 14, "Belly turns out is still constipation so bulking agent! Worked like devils removing old carpet in the attic and Jane scrubbing in the bathroom" (Personal diary, 26 June 2011). The reassurance of the visit to the doctor seems to galvanise and energise us both. The flat needs a great deal of work including complete redecoration and a new kitchen but things are far from being right with Jane.

VA: I was just remembering that time, wanting desperately to fix her and knowing that it was way beyond anything I could fix or even that anybody else could fix. This wasn't good and beyond that I didn't think, I thought about the flat instead.
INTERVIEWER: Okay, this is the difficult bit, there's a bit of a tremble and I just want to say that I'm noticing that.
VA: It was just this thing I think we both knew but didn't consciously acknowledge and certainly beyond saying that it would all be better when we got to Edinburgh, once we could, she just wanted to get into the flat. She just wanted to be in her own place, she wanted to be at home, in her home.

(Interview One, 9 July 2013)

It is the most bittersweet time; we both seem to know but we can neither acknowledge nor admit to ourselves or each other that she may be seriously ill:

She was in a state of tension and it was magnified by her own physical discomfort but also her psychological discomfort of not being at home. So even though the flat was in a fairly ghastly mess, it was light, it was bright, it was airy, it stunk of cigarette smoke but that didn't matter, it was ours, it was a home and we were very quickly going to make it into a little nest that she would feel comfortable in.

(Interview One, 9 July 2013)

Given the poor state of Jane's health, this emphasis on 'being at home' may seem odd. Yet until she felt 'at home' she would not be able to let go and be ill. This was a liminal state, a transition between our previous journeying through Europe, to a home from home at Jane's maternal home, to the sense of permanence that one feels at home. I was unaware just how powerful a concept home was for Jane until I came to reflect upon it for the study. When we worked together in our home-based consultancy she had the habit at the end of the working day of announcing to the house that 'she was home from her work' when all she had done was walk from her study into the kitchen. While I can recognise that I like being at home, prefer to work from home and when away, like to get home, this was something more. Alsop (2002) although writing about studying away from home, discusses the difference between two German terms from which the English word *home* is derived. These are *Heim*, simply home as we understand it in its various contexts, and *Heimat* which has a much more polarised sense of "the rather awful prospect of living in a desert of the familiar, the same; at the other extreme it is a jewel, a gem, something special and very dear and precious to you" (Alsop, 2002: 2).

It was the latter that mattered for Jane. *Heimat* was also a German television mini-series which we had watched a few years ago – all 32 episodes totalling 53 hours. Set in the Hunsrück it detailed life in west Germany from 1919 to 2000. When I had asked Jane then what 'Heimat' meant, she explained that in a simple sense it means 'homeland' but in reality it is far more as she said in her later blog post.[1] The security of our sense of homeland allows an inner compass to develop. We are largely unaware of it until we leave, resulting in a dialectic between home and away, between past and future (Alsop, 2002). When we are away from home we make sense of where we are by continually referencing it in terms of how it might be at home. Much of this may simply be a subconscious process of adapting to our new surroundings. Sometimes we may wish to escape Alsop's 'desert of the familiar' in a rejection of Western culture and capitalism, as part of an existential becoming (Madison, 2006). Jane needed not just to be at home but also to lose the sense of homelessness from the months of travelling and to recover a sense of settled comfort. The idea of homelessness can be further extended to an interpretation of illness where one does not feel at home with one's body. Drawing on Heidegger's conception of *Unheimlichkeit* (uncanniness or unhomelikeness), Svenaeus proposes that this is the essence of illness when:

the mission of health care professionals must consequently be not only to cure diseases, but actually, through devoting attention to the being-in-the-world of the patient, also to open up possible paths back to homelikeness.

(Svenaeus, 2003: 14)

For Jane, unhomelikeness now extended from not being physically at home, to feelings of not being at home in her body. We are about to discover that illness will compound her sense of unhomelikeness. In times of crisis or personal difficulty I tend to resort to black humour as illustrated in an email to my sister in Canada:

We are off again tomorrow for one night with a van to take some big stuff through. Queenie continues to await the arrival of the Royal relief and is now enjoying a fourth type of easing medicine which I have likened to the bomb disposal unit but they seem to be away on manoeuvres. She has been nine months up the duff for a fortnight and won't say who's responsible. So I am hoping a rattly run through in a van might dislodge something.

(Personal email, 3 July 2011)

The humour, which referenced the family joke of 'royal status',[2] was partly to allay my sister's concerns. But it was also an attempt to reinforce a belief in myself that it really was just constipation. The preparations for our new home are a useful distraction but the conspiracy of silence continues and has widened to include other close family members, especially my sister. Perhaps most telling is Jane's silence. She remains stoical and uncomplaining but by day 21, a week after the initial consultation with the new GP, she is in considerable pain. At night she paces up and down, unable to sleep or find relief from the pain and her giant, distended abdomen. We have a night in a nearby hotel in preparation for further flat arrangements. In the morning I make her an urgent appointment at the surgery:

The second time we went to the GP, it was the same chap, the charming young registrar but this time he had a female medical student with him. We had gone into the consulting room and I'd helped her up onto the couch and he'd prodded and looked at this belly and then said that this was an interesting case and he'd like the medical student to examine her as well. What he was showing the medical student was that it was a very good example of profound abdominal ascites and you could do the wave test where you tap on one side and you can see the ripple effect across the abdomen. Jane was always in teaching mode or education mode or learning mode so if there was an opportunity to learn something, and she was a centre of attention in that way, then that made it okay, she could then intellectualise [it as] being interesting. So she could disassociate herself from this was her body that something clearly was going very wrong with. She could then almost be out of it and look at it as an interesting case and join in with the intellectual discussion.

(Interview One, 9 July 2013)

It is perhaps understandable that as Jane had previously been examined and x-rayed in hospital, that following the first GP visit, the diagnosis of constipation continued to be accepted as correct. I found it very difficult to understand this apparent body blindness to what seemed so obvious. The willingness to accept the initial diagnosis and not to see Jane's whole body disfiguration with her thin arms and huge abdomen was at best puzzling. Was this another conspiracy or just simple inexperience in a recently qualified community physician? A paradoxical explanation could be the notion of 'diagnostic creep'. The term was first used in relation to childhood problems of living when it was used to describe them as mental disorders (Anand & Malhi, 2011) and codified by the American Psychiatric Association (Farah, 2002). In the USA, in particular, the term now has some variations:

> Treatment creep is adding new medications without stopping the old. Diagnostic creep comes from multiple diagnoses with medications for each. Doctor creep involves patients securing drugs from multiple providers. Most iatrogenic is Pharma creep with a pill for every human unhappiness.
> (Brendtro & Mitchell, 2013: 7)

Effects of this 'creep' can include a willingness to accept a diagnosis once it has been made or to overdiagnose; a result of wider definitions of disease and earlier detection (Moynihan et al., 2012). Doctors are trained to act, symbolised in general practice by the prescription which may be unlikely to make any real difference to the patient's condition, yet there is "a pill for every ill" (Busfield, 2010: 934). For whatever reason, Jane's symptoms of bloating and abdominal discomfort could be accounted for by the earlier diagnosis of constipation. Malignant ascites, the accumulation of fluid in the abdomen as a result of neoplastic disease, only accounts for about 10% of all cases. Of those who do present with ascites, 50% do so at their initial diagnosis (Ayantunde & Parsons, 2007). In fact, abdominal bloating and its associated distension has become so common, one Canadian gastroenterologist has stated:

> most cases of functional abdominal bloating with visible abdominal distention can be explained by some combination of weak or inappropriately relaxed abdominal muscles, a diaphragm that contracts when it should relax; excessive intra-abdominal fat; fluid in loops of small intestine and gravity.
> (Sullivan, 2012: 1)

However, something more serious is suggested at our second visit to the surgery.

I had taken to actively guarding Jane, being a layer of protection to fend people off who might collide with her and bump into her because moving around was difficult. If she got jarred or shoved then that was really excruciating so I had this way of walking slightly in front of her with my arm out to deflect anyone. That kind of protection extended into other things as well, I would guard her from whoever needed to see her or to examine her. So the GP says that he's concerned this is clearly more than constipation and that he wants to refer her to the surgical receiving [unit]. So he writes the referral letter and we have to go there.

[At the hospital] I help her get into a gown and up on the trolley and a young male doctor comes in and wants to examine her. I'm sitting on a chair but I stand up and say 'hang on a minute who are you and what is it you're doing'? He sort of jumps back and says 'oh he's sorry, he's doctor'.[3] So I said 'well that's fine' and I'm going to stay with her if that's okay with him and we agree that it is. He examines her abdomen and then does various internal examinations. Doctors learn very early on to have that kind of dead pan expression but I know that this is more and Jane knows but she is relying on me to protect her. So there's a lot of eye contact between us and I'm making lots of reassuring noises.

(Interview One, 9 July 2013)

A 'posse' of doctors return with a plan: Jane needs an ultrasound and a referral to the gynaecologists who are based at another hospital on the other side of the city. The ultrasound cannot be done until the next day. There is then some prevarication about whether she should be admitted that afternoon or allowed to go home; our transport was still the hired van which had to be returned. I negotiate going home, despite the 100 mile round trip.

We want to go back to Glasgow tonight because of course she wants to go home. So we get this agreement that yes she can go home but we will come back through for nine o'clock the following morning for the ultrasound to be done so I have asserted her right to do as she wishes which is to go home.

(Interview One, 9 July 2013)

The inter-hospital referral letter summarises the situation:

Thank you for seeing this 50 year old lady so quickly in your clinic. She presented to us with a history of constipation and a distended abdomen gradually getting worse for the past 2 months. She gave a history of generalised mild abdominal tenderness as well, with no real distinguishing features. She also complained of the occasional feeling of lethargy. ... The impression is of a possible cervical lesion with an unknown cause for her ascites and we would appreciate your urgent opinion regarding this.

(Hospital letter, 5 July 2011)

In the evening, I note in my diary:

Phoned GP this morning and went to see him. Clearly concerned and referred to surgeons. They thought they could feel something so referred to gynae.

Can go back to Glasgow tonight but have to be back for scan at 9am. Worry makes the world go round.

(Personal diary, 5 July 2011)

Although it is not mentioned in either my diary or the more recent interview, I also remember driving back via the flat and parking so we were facing the building. We sat looking at our new home, reassuring ourselves that all would be fine once we could get into the flat and just be there with our two cats. We agree to try and be brave and wait for the outcome of the ultrasound the following day. The drive back to Glasgow was a quiet run, neither of us saying much. Whatever is wrong with Jane, we are certain that as she is otherwise fit and healthy, we will be equal to any challenges.

Finding

In this episode, the cause of Jane's symptoms is discovered following an emergency hospital admission and a provisional diagnosis of advanced ovarian cancer is made. It begins with an unsettled night for us both then the drive back to Edinburgh where we report to reception at the specialist centre for reproductive health. My memories remain vivid as I recall the procedure:

> We were told to wait in an area for ultrasound but what was very strange and I think what was very difficult for her, was that the unit in the hospital is both for women with gynaecological disorders but also for women who are pregnant. So most of the ultrasounds and certainly all of the other women that were waiting were obviously pregnant and Jane looked both older and whilst at first glance she might have looked pregnant, she also didn't look right. The radiographer was on one side and I sat on the other and they started doing the ultrasound. Quite quickly the radiographer could see there was a mass and she started measuring it and called to her colleague. They were talking about 12 cms. I was making reassuring noises but we were just kind of exchanging looks that said yes there is something.
>
> *(Interview Two, 13 August 2013)*

Following the ultrasound we are ushered by a senior nurse to a side room with a hospital bed. Later I learnt this is a triage area for gynaecological emergencies. A woman in theatre scrubs comes to explain the surgeon is in theatre but he will come as soon as he was free. Something has changed, I can see it in the nurse's face, nothing is too much trouble, the situation has shifted, this really is serious.

VA: Eventually [the surgeon] came and was very smiley and charming and asked Jane all sorts of questions about her medical history and how long this had been going on for. Then he wanted to do an internal examination but she was in an extremely uncomfortable position and when he tried to examine her, it was excruciatingly painful. He didn't really try very hard and just sort of said no, it was okay, he would leave it. What he really needed to do was to take her to theatre and do a diagnostic laparoscopy to see what was going on. He could get her into the end of the list that day and so that was the plan but she needed to go and have a chest x-ray. Then we were sitting waiting and suddenly the surgeon reappeared and said right, that was it, he was ready for her and he whisked her off upstairs. There wasn't anything else I could do, there was no point in me waiting, I just had to leave.

INTERVIEWER: How was she when she heard she was going to have to go to theatre that day?

VA: Oh, she was excited, she'd seemed quite small a lot of the time. If I say she was almost child-like, I don't mean that in a derogatory sense but there was this kind of wide-eyed innocence and part of that wide-eyed innocence was curiosity to what was going on, what was happening. She hadn't ever spent a night in hospital all her life. I think it was almost part of her coping mechanism to ignore the fact that it was her body that was being looked at and poked and prodded and examined. This was something exciting that was happening. Her father had been a laboratory technician and so she had that sort of medical curiosity of what's going on. Wanting to know and I suppose consoling herself with what her dad would have thought of it and how she would tell him all about it.

(Interview Two, 13 August 2013)

I remember walking away from the hospital to spend the first night in the flat alone and phoning her mother to explain something had been found and that a small, exploratory operation was needed. We both had difficulty speaking, neither one wanting to acknowledge what we both feared. Any conspiracy of silence had gone, replaced by a state of fearfulness. Denial of serious illness is a complex concept that originated in psychotherapeutic practice with patients who had difficulty in accepting what had happened to their bodies. It can range on a continuum through non-acceptance of diagnosis, minimising the seriousness of their condition, delay in seeking help, poor compliance with treatment and appearing to have an unperturbed detachment with regard to their illness (Goldbeck, 1997). It may be perceived by health professionals as either an ineffective defence mechanism or as an adaptive strategy for coping with overwhelming feelings and events (Vos & Haes, 2007). For Jane, and indeed for me and her mother, there had been a denial of illness but privately we all had our suspicions. It was only when the bodily illness could no longer be concealed that its presence is accepted. A diagnosis of cancer is anticipated by all three of us; denial had been a temporary adaptive strategy.

It is three weeks before Jane writes a blog post about what has happened. Then she tells the whole story starting with the journey back from London, the constipation diagnosis and the laparoscopy, to the first chemotherapy session. Consequently, in order to include her version of events, the chronology is slightly distorted as is the tenor of her voice. She is upbeat, humorous, her usual witty self but by the time of writing, she knew the extent of the disease and the treatment plan. She sets the scene at the outset, acknowledging the delay and her intended purpose in writing.

> Our little world turned upside down and it's taken a wee while before I've felt able to write about what's been happening. In short: I've been diagnosed with ovarian cancer. Now I really do not want the account of our lives and journeys I've been keeping here to turn into 'yet another cancer blog'. What follows is rather long, and quite personal, perhaps too personal, and with too much information for some. But there's nothing like having cancer to illuminate starkly what really matters in life, removing prevarication, inhibition and equivocation. It gives focus, makes you honest, strips you bare.
>
> (Blog post 'Silver Linings', 28 July 2011)

The authenticity of her account following this blunt introduction is accurate, almost as if she had a video recording of the proceedings. This may be accounted for by the heightened awareness experienced in times of anxiety through the fight or flight response (Cannon, 1932). Barbara Rosenblum described how her training as a sociologist made her acutely aware of the demeanour of her doctor during their first clinical encounter, "I searched for clues to anticipate what she would tell me" (Butler & Rosenblum, 1991: 10). I had recognised something similar in the way Jane comported herself in hospital as I recall in the interview excerpt above "that wide-eyed innocence was curiosity to what was going on, what was happening" (Interview Two, 13 August 2013). That wide-eyed curiosity is apparent in her description of the ultrasound and other investigative procedures.

> The following morning I reported for an ultrasound and it was pretty clear from the picture, and the whispered conversations ('I can't find the left ovary', 'Just take measurements then') that there was indeed something unpleasant in my pelvic area. The gynae consultant came down, tried to do an internal, pronounced himself 'confused' by what he'd found, and admitted me for exploratory surgery. I had an examination under anaesthetic and a diagnostic laparoscopy later that afternoon (the consultant having gone to some lengths to make space in the schedule, and to persuade the anaesthetist to admit me to theatre without his usual checks – 'My colleague assures me you are strong and fit and a suitable candidate for surgery, so I'm just going to knock you out now.')
>
> Then I got to spend my first ever night in hospital, and the following morning had an MRI scan and CT scan. Both fascinating procedures: the CT scan a huge spinning wheel of lasers issuing breathing instructions in a vaguely amusing mid-Atlantic accent; the MRI scan that big scary washing machine thing that swallows you whole served up on a metal tray. I overcame any sense of claustrophobia by pretending to be Sigourney Weaver settling down

for the trip back to Earth at the end of Alien (not entirely inappropriate given the enemy currently consuming me from within). I accepted the offer of classical music for the 25 minutes the scan was to last. Should have had money on the playlist: Pachelbel's *Canon*, Albinoni's *Adagio*, Barber's *Adagio for Strings*, Rachmaninov's *1st Piano Concerto* … all good relaxing stuff if you like funereal music.

(Blog post 'Silver Linings', 28 July 2011)

The trope most apparent to me in this extract is the use of irony, although it will be less obvious to a reader who had not known Jane. Initially, by quoting the overheard comments, she gives an ironic slant to the proceedings, as if the health care professionals appear befuddled by her curious case. She then shifts to using wistful metaphor in her recollection of Sigourney Weaver as the heroic Amazon who has slain the demonic alien. In her mind's eye she recalls the image of a slim, lithe and calm woman (her ideal type) resting quietly in her sleeping pod on her voyage back to Earth. In a review of the Alien trilogy, Murphy makes some interesting observations pertinent to the study, the first being on the concept of home:

> In the nothingness of outer space, the integrity and particularity of flesh is everything. Home is literally where the heart is – the body being the last bastion of warm, colourful, imperfect, familiar biology in a totally deracinating environment.
>
> *(Murphy, 1992: 17)*

Here the irony becomes apparent, as Jane finds solace in her own warm body it is also in full awareness of the alien presence within. For now she can take refuge, but in her disembodied state she hears 'funereal music', a portent of what lies ahead, beyond this liminal place. But her focus will have been on the memory of her heroine, she is yet beautiful:

> And the celebratory inventory of the elegant lines of Ripley's torso and her long, bare arms and legs mark precisely Alien's mortal stakes. These fleshly signatures underscore the strength and beauty of the human body, differentiating it from the alien anatomy.
>
> *(Murphy, 1992: 18)*

The real irony is if Jane had been asked to name four pieces of classical music she most disliked, she would have named the four played in the scanner. The calming and well-intentioned music will have been a grating irritation and anything but relaxing. Lambek (2003) has suggested that there are two forms of irony pertinent to illness: irony of commission or intentional, and irony of recognition or found. It is reasonable to assume that there was no deliberate intention on the part of the technician to play what some might perceive as funereal music. However, it could be classed as an example of irony of recognition: Jane not only recognises the music being played but also its associations in other contexts. Lambek (2003: 1) suggests that "therapeutic practices and discourses can be described and distinguished according to the degree to which they recognise or refuse irony". In this regard I believe it was simply an innocent lack of awareness of music as a powerful synaesthetic agent (Campen, 2014).

Later,[4] when we talk about the episode and by way of preparation for the many scans she will have, I ask if she is going to mention the music and propose something from her own playlist. She thinks not; she would not want to make a fuss or draw attention to herself. This reticence was unusual as previously if something was not to her liking she would have said as much but now it seems it is either less important or the effort is too much. She can make a fuss within the privacy of her own home but does not want to be exposed in the public, clinical space. A more likely explanation is that of feeling powerless at the enormity of her diagnosis (Sand et al., 2008). If we are to believe the veracity of the blog post, 'Silver Linings', the diagnosis was a shock, but Jane does not appear powerless. One interpretation of powerlessness is to view it as something from which empowerment, with features of self-awareness and self-determination, can evolve (Aujoulat et al., 2007). Furthermore "the notion of empowerment should therefore extend to decisions such as the decision to hand over one's responsibility for disease and treatment, provided the decision is sufficiently informed and self-determined" (Aujoulat et al., 2007: 772).

This seems a more plausible explanation; there is little Jane can *do*, she just has to endure procedures, treatment or even ubiquitous music. It is human nature to assume an active role in response to any given situation but this may not always be possible or appropriate. Jane understood this through her understanding of Goethe's synthesis of thinking and doing (Plenderleith, 1993). She is content to swap *doing* for *being*, passively thinking and absorbing all that happens around and to her. This dialectic process is a process of becoming (Wilcock, 1999), a transition from who she thought herself to be, to who she is now becoming.

The next day I want to go to the hospital as soon as possible but Jane calls to say she is fine; I should wait until lunchtime when the doctor will explain what has been found. In the second interview, I am asked what Jane might prepare herself for.

> I don't know at what point she must have realised. Actually I think she knew when they did the ultrasound because we both knew that there was a large tumour and so then what she was preparing herself for was how they were going to get rid of this thing and make her better. She was quite upbeat, they had found something and they'd taken the biopsies. The next step was to be seen by the oncologist and then if they were able to shrink the tumour, the surgeon would then be able to remove it. So, although the news was devastating, there was a positive plan.
>
> *(Interview Two, 13 August 2013)*

There are further tests to be done before she can leave but finally we are given a discharge letter for the GP and a supply of a cloyingly sweet high protein drink. This is to counter the loss of albumin from when the ascites was drained in theatre. I read the discharge letter and see words that burn my eyes "peritoneum obliterated by disease, widespread miliary disease in pelvis, pelvic organs stuck, tumour in omentum. Not surgically resectable. Diaphragms covered, porta involved" (Hospital discharge letter, 6 July 2011).

A distant horizon brings the word *carcinomatosis* and the thirty year old memory of a woman, a teacher in her early fifties, with luminous, foul-smelling liquid oozing from her bloated abdomen. I was a student nurse, horrified by the sight, the stench and her suffering. The famous line from Wilfred Owen's (1920) *Dulce et Decorum Est*, "Gas! Gas! Quick, boys! – An ecstasy of fumbling" is apposite as I recall the bedside scene. It was the second year of my nurse training but still I fumbled in embarrassment for fear of showing my revulsion. Then the woman in her sixties, when I was a third year on night duty, with the fistula between her vagina and rectum constantly leaking foul-smelling liquid. I did not speak of these horrors; Jane cannot understand why I am so upset. She is content with the plan as presented. I am thankful she does not realise that *miliary disease* means the primary tumour had already 'bloomed' and secondary, metastatic disease has spread within her abdomen. I now realise that if the disease had not been found then, she would probably have died within a few weeks. The ultrasound report[5] confirms the off-stage whispers we had heard during the procedure:

> Technically difficult ultrasound examination. The uterus and left ovary was not visualised. There is a solid and cystic mass extending from the right side of the pelvis to the left, this is highly suspicious of a right sided ovarian malignancy. The mass measures approximately 92x56x75mm. Significant free fluid noted in the pelvis and abdomen.
>
> *(Ultrasound report, 6 July 2011)*

I note in my diary "the doctor came and confirmed our worst fears ... bit shell shocked" (Personal diary, 7 July 2011). Terror management theory (TMT) is a useful way for clinicians to interpret their anxieties when they feel a patient may be in denial of serious illness (Rayson, 2013). TMT was first proposed in the 1980s (Greenberg et al., 1986) and based on Ernest Becker's idea that most human action is taken to avoid or ignore death. TMT is centred on self-esteem as an essential mechanism that acts as a buffer against existential anxiety. The terror of our own death is ameliorated by how good we feel about ourselves. The sense of personal value extends to a sense of how we might 'live on' after physical death in either a literal or symbolic sense. Belief in an afterlife or heaven provides literal relief of death anxiety while having children or particular life achievements affords symbolic relief (Burke et al., 2010). Rayson summarises TMT in the context of palliation as "Our patients know the end is coming. We know the end is coming. We all need to keep on keeping on" (Rayson, 2013: 4372).

Now we both know the end is coming, yet Jane's horizon is two years. She believes and has complete faith in the proposed treatment plan. This is consistent with the finding that cancer patients are much more interested and focused on treatment than on prognosis (Salander, 2002). It is also consistent with the earlier insight from TMT where Jane's courage and energy can be deployed in feeling good, despite the news. There is treatment available and she will try her best. However, the news of her illness now needs to be broadcast to our immediate family.

INTERVIEWER: So that night, she phoned and told her sisters. How did she prepare herself to do that?

VA: Well, we'd driven back and told her mother. I think in telling her mother, as a linguist Jane was very good at rehearsing what she wanted to say and so it didn't really matter whether she was going say it in French or German or in English, she would rehearse. She would have rehearsed in her head what she was going to say and the way in which the news would be presented. So yes, there was bad news but there was a positive message that the surgeon had taken biopsies and the oncologist would then know what kind of chemotherapy to use. The tumour would shrink and the surgeon would then remove it. So it was very much presented as a complete package without any kind of question that maybe the tumour wouldn't respond or the surgeon might not be able to remove it or that even surgery might not be such a good idea because of the other things that it might entail.

(Interview Two, 13 August 2013)

As with Schaepe's (2011) finding that the diagnosis may be conveyed incrementally by different clinicians until the ultimate meeting with the oncologist, so it is for Jane. At this point the information is equivocal, nothing would or could be confirmed until the pathology report is received and the oncologist is able to determine the precise type of chemotherapy to use. Questions regarding prognosis do not arise; it is enough to try and understand the provisional diagnosis. However, in a systematic review of conveying cancer prognosis, Hagerty et al. (2005) recognised the desire of patients to be more involved in the decision-making process regarding their care and treatment. But the emphasis is on the best method of communicating prognosis based on patient preferences. The enormity of that first 24 hours is evident in my diary entry the following day:

So many tears shed in the last 24hrs but J incredibly brave and stoical. She told [her sisters] last night and I phoned [my sister]. Today we just tried to get our heads around the basics and will now get decorators to do flat.

(Personal diary, 8 July 2011)

In the interview excerpt I say "as a linguist Jane was very good at rehearsing what she wanted to say" which encapsulates the essence of the unfolding drama in which we now found ourselves. The first definition of a linguist is a person skilled in languages, and the second is someone who speaks freely and eloquently (*SOED*, 2007). Jane had both of these attributes. Part of her rehearsal process is not just to work out in her mind the correct words and grammar to use but also to tell it in a pleasing way. So there is bad news, cancer, but this is quickly assuaged with good news, treatment plan, all packaged in a few succinct and eloquent sentences. Of course her mother already knows when she is told, as mothers do, for she has noticed Jane's 'scrawny neck'. I am not surprised she realised there was something seriously wrong with her daughter, nor that she joined in the conspiracy of silence. The dissemination of the news becomes easier for Jane as she works her way down through the layers of family, friends and work colleagues she wants to tell. Stacey considers the effect on relationships as she describes the process for each outsider as they gain this insider knowledge:

> A complex interchange of projection and protection is at play in this process of sharing the news. Has so-and-so heard? How did they react? And through their shocked reaction your own sense of discrepancy between who-you-thought-you-were and who-you-must-now-be is repeatedly rehearsed.
>
> *(Stacey, 1997: 70)*

The dance has started and the first few steps set the scene for how the entire dance will play out. The process for selecting the corps de ballet to support the two principals is underway. The company quickly self-selects itself as those family members and friends, who for whatever reason do not want to join the dance, slip away. Curiously as the news spreads, long lost friends reappear and join the dance, staying to the end. The reactions of others to the news is not lost on Jane either:

> Other people react to my cancer in interesting ways. Some stay away, not, I think, in case they catch something nasty, but simply because they don't know what to say. Mostly people rally round. We take huge comfort from the overwhelming waves of love and support and concern, popping in to say hello, the phone calls, emails and texts that just stay in touch and say 'we care', the offers to help in any way possible. I'm figuring in the prayers of a lot of people including the Iona prayer group (special because Iona is special to us, where serenity meets energy). I'll take all the help I can get. Francophones send courage. [A cousin's daughter] wrote 'Dad and I were just saying if anyone can beat this, Jane can'. That sort of ringing endorsement does a power of good.
>
> *(Blog post 'Silver Linings', 28 July 2011)*

My own role is already heroic, Amazon carer.

> What I didn't want because I knew, my imagination was running away with all the things that she was going have to face, but I didn't want her to be fearful. I wanted her to feel safe and as protected as possible, that she wasn't alone and we'd make it as easy as we could. She wasn't to fear that she would be in pain or that it would be too horrid or whatever, that it would be okay.

That was right from the diagnosis, that was hugely important, that I was there and with her all the way.

(Interview Two, 13 August 2013)

In the telling of the news she is perhaps doing as Butler and Rosenblum (1991) suggest and not just communicating her difficult situation but also recruiting supporters to her cause. This is in part confirmed by an email from my sister "it felt good to feel the circle of love and connection between us all … the pair of you mean the world to us" (Personal email, 12 July 2011).

We waste no time during the week between the diagnostic laparoscopy and the first appointment with the oncologist, in getting Jane into training for the challenge ahead. She rests with her very oedematous legs elevated, drinks the saccharine protein drinks and generally takes life easy. I rush about like a woman possessed, which of course I am, continually haunted by dark thoughts, and fuss over Jane to her mild irritation. The culmination of my experience as a nurse with some insight into gynaecological cancers and expertise in the care of the dying have the makings of a *return enhanced*. Lay carers may have feelings of uncertainty and a lack of rehearsal when preparing to care for a partner or relative with advanced illness (Newbury, 2009). A sense of disruption and unpreparedness is evident in the artist Marion Coutts' first-hand account of caring for her husband with glioma (Coutts, 2014). As I prepare to care for Jane, I do not have these feelings, nor have I lost my sense of self by becoming bound to Jane's dependent body (Jenkinson, 2004). I care for Jane's body but it is not the body I know in intimate detail, for that seems to have gone forever after her sojourn in hospital; replaced by a bloated and disfigured shape as a semblance of her former self.

We return to Edinburgh for the first night in the flat sans furniture apart from a studio couch. I make an impromptu recliner for Jane with a camping chair and a discarded stool. We sit in the window looking at the view of the Pentland Hills and the clouds, on the edge of excitement. The meeting with the oncologist is the following morning when the great plan will be revealed.

Planning

In the last story of this chapter, we attend the first clinic appointment with the oncologist, learn the outcome of the pathology report and the forward plan for Jane's care. There are three different accounts of the meeting, first my interview recollection is intended to set the ethnographic scene. Then the oncologist's medical case note provides confirmation and finally Jane's blog post is the dance director's version for public broadcast. The appointment is at the same hospital Jane attended when referred by her GP. It is also where I was a ward sister and a night charge nurse in what was then the radiotherapy unit and is now the regional cancer centre.

> The clinic itself was a relatively small area but what I really remember was that there were a lot of women there already, maybe six or so and they all had

somebody with them. They all looked just pained and anxious and some were quite tearful. There was an absolutely palpable tension; we were told to sit down and wait. I'd taken the iPad because as long as Jane had something to distract her that was fine. It had the *Guardian* on it and also puzzles so she could just hold that and lose herself in something and not be drawn in to this tension. But the staff were doing their best, there was a staff nurse who was checking people's weights and Jane's turn came for that.

Eventually it was her turn to be seen and this youngish chap came and we were ushered into a consulting room. It was one of those dreich wee places that's just literally a desk, a couple of chairs and an examination couch. We sat down and we'd rehearsed some of what we might say. We understood that this wasn't good news, it was quite serious. There was the plan was to try chemotherapy first and hope that the tumour shrank and then it could be removed. I did a lot of the talking but tried to make sure that Jane got to say what she wanted to say but I remember emphasising that we were educationalists, that the way we dealt with things was to see what could be learnt from them and that if there was any research being done or if there were medical students that wanted to examine Jane or anything like that at all then that was absolutely not a problem, Jane was very keen. So he explained that yes, the pathology results were that it was a serous cell tumour and the staging was 3C which is not quite the worst; the plan would be to start chemotherapy. Then he said he would try and see if he could get her into the chemotherapy unit to start treatment the following day.

We went back out into the waiting area and it felt like this huge relief because treatment was going to start as soon as possible and that meant a huge amount to Jane. Although this had taken a long time to find out, as soon as they knew they were going to react as quickly as they could. So although there was still this tension, these unhappy women sitting there, she was almost smiling because she was going to be fixed. Then he came back and said yes indeed, he'd managed to get her in, they would do some bloods and there were pills that needed to be taken the night before. So that was it and off we went, almost excited.

(Interview Three, 20 August 2013)

Once again a performance has been rehearsed and given in a private audience. I am carried along by Jane's enthusiasm for quick action, her complete faith in the Scottish NHS and some private pride that *my* hospital is preparing to give her the best treatment available. The oncologist summarises his findings in a letter sent to the GP:

> The lady has a Grade 3 Stage 3C serous papillary ovarian carcinoma. It is clear that this has progressed rapidly and the extent of the disease is considerable. We had a discussion about the aims and side effect of Carboplatin and Paclitaxel chemotherapy. The lady and her partner were already well up to speed with

the situation and the precarious situation that she is in. I felt that in view of the rapid progression of the disease that we had to initiate chemotherapy straight away and therefore I have arranged for the lady to receive her first cycle of chemotherapy tomorrow. She will receive 3 cycles of 3 weekly chemotherapy and then immediately after this will have a CT scan so we can consider whether interval debulking is a possibility. The lady knows from her consultation today that this is very far from certain as the extent of her disease makes surgery a very big undertaking indeed.

(Hospital case records cover sheet, 14 July 2011)

The oncologist's account confirms we gave a reasonable performance and conveys our genuine understanding of Jane's situation. He really wants to help, to see if there is the slimmest chance that the tumour will shrink and that surgery will be possible. But Jane did not seem to hear that "this is very far from certain as the extent of her disease". What she focused on was that treatment would start the following day, immediately. But then it is clear from the following blog extract that she has heard and understood a great deal of what was said and the reality of her situation.

It's a bit of a facer when your world turns upside down and everything you've planned for, everything you thought was important, suddenly and seismically shifts. The full diagnosis was revealed by my lovely young oncologist (yes there is a pattern here, I am surrounded by lovely young highly intelligent capable professionals) the following week. Here it is.

I have a Stage 3 serous tumour which started on my left ovary (or fallopian tube, there's some debate), has munched its way through most of my uterus and 'involves' (they're not sure of the extent) the bladder wall and the rectum. It has also pressed on the ureter to the extent that my left kidney has stopped functioning. Treatment is to be four cycles of chemotherapy in the first instance, which they hope will shrink the tumour to an operable size, then a hysterectomy. He said that [the surgeon] has told him they are going to have to do 'a really good job with the chemo' and that is exactly what they are trying to do. I'm not sure how he did it, he had to move a few mountains or sell his soul or both, but he persuaded the cancer day unit to admit me for my first chemo session the following day. Officially, then, from diagnosis to chemotherapy in less than 24 hours – I will never again hear a bad word about our NHS.

Our meeting with [the oncologist] was really interesting. He started with his concerned 'I'm sorry to tell you you've got cancer' face and tone of voice, closely followed by what is apparently the next worst thing he can tell you, 'now you will lose your hair … but we can give you a wig!'. But when we reassured him that this news was not entirely unexpected, that we'd had a pretty good idea of the size and shape of things to come when we'd left the hospital the week before, had got our heads round things, and no thank you I did not want a wig, his whole tone and demeanour changed. He went through my family health history in some detail, suggesting that there may be a genetic trigger for ovarian cancer in one so young as me (hah!). We wanted him to know that we're in this together, that I have huge support at home (practical, clinical and emotional), that we are really positive about the treatment, will do all we can to maximise its effectiveness, and have every confidence in the team that's looking after me at Edinburgh, that we have an intellectual as well as personal interest in what's going on, a lifelong concern with education and research, and that I am more than happy to be a teaching case or participate in medical trials. [The oncologist's] particular interest is genetic causes of ovarian cancer and he has stored some of my blood for possible DNA testing[6] as part of his research at a later date (if and when he can persuade the government to fund an extension to his study).

(Blog post 'Silver Linings', 28 July 2011)

Following the diagnosis and meeting with the oncologist, neither of us is inclined to search for information on the internet or read booklets from support agencies such as Macmillan. I download the SIGN (Scottish Intercollegiate Guidelines Network) *Guidelines for the Management of Epithelial Ovarian Cancer* (2003) but do not discuss the details with Jane. I just want to refresh my understanding of the disease and to confirm she will be getting the best treatment available. These summary points seem relevant to my understanding of Jane's situation (SIGN, 2003: 1):

- Ovarian cancer is the fourth most frequently diagnosed cancer in women in Scotland, representing 4.6% of all newly diagnosed cancers, or around 600 new cases per year in Scotland.
- The aetiology of the disease is unknown and is more common in women who have never been pregnant.
- Among women in Scotland with no family history, the lifetime risk of developing ovarian cancer is estimated to be 1 in 59.
- Survival is dependent on the stage of cancer at initial presentation – whilst stage I disease has a five year survival rate of 85%, stage IV disease has a five year survival rate of only approximately 10%.
- Epithelial ovarian cancer is described as a 'silent killer' as in over 60% of cases advanced disease is found at initial presentation.
- The goal for health professionals must be to ensure that where cure is not possible a woman can have a good quality of life with judicious use of surgery and chemotherapy.

My clinical curiosity is overwhelmed by the stark confirmation of the evidence; the outlook for Jane is not good. Most of the terms I hear being discussed or read in the discharge letter, I know and understand apart from 'neoadjuvant chemotherapy'. It came into medical parlance in the 1990s to indicate the use of systemic treatment, either chemical or radiation, prior to local surgical intervention particularly in cases of solid tumours (Trimble et al., 1993). Its use in our context is entirely consistent but some have proposed:

> Terminology in medicine should be lucid, understandable, consistent and unambiguous. The technical meaning of each term should correspond closely to what is generally understood by ordinary people, thus excluding confusion between patients, clinicians and researchers.
>
> *(Habbema et al., 2004: 1499)*

This may seem a little strong given that we do understand most of what is said and the health care professionals are also aware of my nursing background. Nevertheless there is a continuing tendency to use highly specialised medical language with the assumption that its understanding is unnecessary for the general public, despite the increasing use of the internet as patients try to understand their medical conditions and treatment regimes. Awareness of new treatments and active research trials is openly encouraged by charities such as Cancer Research UK who provide a comprehensive website[7] with easy access to information regarding current trials. It is claimed by Cancer Research UK that more people in the UK participate in trials than anywhere else in the world. The guidelines on epithelial ovarian cancer were updated in 2013[8] and the revised version makes some additional points regarding the detection of ovarian cancer in primary care (SIGN, 2013):

- Retrospective studies show that women with ovarian cancer present with non-specific symptoms including abdominal pain and bloating, changes in bowel habit, urinary and/or pelvic symptoms.
- Cachexia (weakness and wasting due to serious illness) is uncommon and women with advanced disease often look surprisingly well.
- Most women with ovarian cancer are diagnosed when they already have advanced disease.
- On average, a GP will see only one new case every five years (Hamilton, 2012).
- Patients who present with non-specific gastrointestinal symptoms may be misdiagnosed as suffering from irritable bowel syndrome.

Ovarian cancer therefore is a relatively rare disease that can present with a variety of vague and confusing symptoms which may have never been seen by the primary care physician. However, in the intervening ten years between publication of the two guidelines there has been a rapid increase in both research into ovarian cancer in general and awareness raising of the most common symptoms. The ovarian cancer charity, Ovacome, launched a campaign in 2010 using the acronym BEAT:[9]

- B for bloating that is persistent and doesn't come and go
- E for eating less and feeling fuller

- A for abdominal pain
- T for telling your GP

In 2011, the National Institute for Health and Clinical Excellence (NICE) published guidelines on the initial recognition of ovarian cancer by clinicians. It recommended that tests should be carried out in primary care on women, especially those over 50, who have any of the following symptoms frequently or persistently, with particular attention to more than 12 occurrences in a month:

1. persistent abdominal distension ('bloating')
2. feeling full (early satiety) and/or loss of appetite
3. pelvic or abdominal pain
4. increased urinary urgency and/or frequency *(NICE, 2011: 10)*

Jane had all of these symptoms and was seen by four different doctors (two men, two women), all in the first few years of their careers,[10] none of whom seemed to recognise a pattern. NICE is an agency that operates in England and Wales but there was also similar information in the first Scottish guideline (SIGN, 2003). It is a commonly held belief that delays in the diagnosis and treatment of cancer have a negative impact on survival yet delays are approximately equal in attribution to both the patient and the GP. Furthermore these delays do not affect survival of ovarian cancer beyond 18 months (Kirwan et al., 2002). The experience of an average general practice in seeing more unusual conditions was described in the 1960s as an illness iceberg, disease which is known to the average clinician but is undetected (Last & Adelaide, 1963). Hannay (1980) developed this idea by contrasting the iceberg of illness with trivial consultations that were bothersome to GPs. He concluded that there were significant symptoms in the community that were not reported to family doctors especially by middle-aged women. The term 'illness behaviour' (Mechanic, 1961) was first used to account for the different ways in which symptoms are perceived and acted upon, including being ignored, by individuals.

The delay in seeking help when faced with some bodily change could also be understood from inner and outer body perspectives. Inwardly there may be recognition of some vague symptom or change in bodily function but to acknowledge it is potentially to take it out into the world, perhaps even to health care. If the change has not been recognised or sanctioned by a family member then it can be even more easily dismissed as something trivial (Smith et al., 2005). Making the shift to understand the true meaning of a bodily disturbance may be a "breakdown in accommodation" (Radley, 2004: 73) and is based on Zola's five 'triggers' to seek medical attention, "an interpersonal crisis, *perceived* interference in relationships, sanctioning when someone else takes the decision, *perceived* interference with physical activity and recurrence or existence of signs over a period of time" (Zola, 1973: 683, original emphasis). In the blog post when she announces her diagnosis, Jane reflects on her awareness of the illness:

> I arrived back in Glasgow on a train from London after a meeting one evening in the middle of June with an aching back (I'd had a sore back for months, which we put down to strange spare beds and the left-hand drive car) and a swollen, painful abdomen. After a couple of sleepless nights we decided something had to be done.
>
> *(Blog post 'Silver Linings', 28 July 2011)*

Here the breakdown of accommodation is the persistence of a symptom over time, 'a sore back for months', and the interference of physical activity, 'after a couple of sleepless nights' that results in action, 'something had to be done'. There is also the suggestion of sanctioning by the use of the plural 'we decided', she had my agreement that help should be sought. Earlier I have suggested there was a conspiracy of silence when Jane appeared to be unwell yet colluded in an unspoken tacit agreement to ignore her situation. I am also aware of an element of bystander apathy, a state of personal indecision and conflict concerning whether to act or not (Latané & Darley, 1969). However, I know that any vacillation on my part did not affect the outcome (Kirwan et al., 2002). There is also little to suggest that investigation any months earlier would have made a difference. In a study of more than 800 ovarian cancer patients "Use of symptoms to trigger medical evaluation for ovarian cancer is likely to result in diagnosis of the disease in only one of 100 women" (Rossing et al., 2010: 222).

It is impossible for me to think of Jane's situation without recalling the women I had cared for in the past: my feelings are completely foregrounded by my past experience. My comfort zone is to try and engage with the clinical aspects of the diagnosis and the treatment; I want to be included in the discussions of the health care team. My dialogic self (Hermans, 2001) needs conversations about what is happening and I cannot discuss clinical details with Jane. I can supply any amount of discrete information and support but not the dark detail of my previous experience. Nor can I begin to imagine how it is for Jane, what she really feels. I deflect direct questions with simple enquires as to how she is doing and that is understood to encompass a myriad of possibilities. Then she gives the public a version of her feelings:

> My reaction to cancer is quite interesting to me too. It's another adventure. Not one we would have chosen to undertake, but it has presented itself and has to be undergone, and overcome, with as much grace and dignity as it's possible to muster. It's also quite an education (a recent article in the *Guardian* expressed the educational aspects of cancer far more elegantly than I can). I don't feel resentment, or fear. I'm not asking the two unanswerable questions, 'why me?' and 'how long have I got?'. I didn't think I was angry but I have been responding with disproportionate fury to slight irritations, so there may be something to work through there … There's nothing like cancer to restore perspective on what really matters in life.
>
> *(Blog post 'Silver Linings', 28 July 2011)*

First she uses her usual upbeat style, turning the experience into one that can be understood through education. The article to which she refers is a personal account of living with multiple myeloma, by the late American author Mike Marqusee. I believe this is what appealed to her:

> But what exactly have I learned? To begin with, that any glib answer to the question misses the core of the experience – the complex dialectic of being ill, which is a social as well as physical condition. For me the experience has led to a heightened awareness of both our intricate dependence on others and our deep-seated need for independence.
>
> (Marqusee, 2011: 1)

She was, as I recall, acutely aware of her dependence on others, not just on me but all of the people involved in her care, her team of health care workers as well as friends and family. What made her angry was not so much the disease itself but the impact on her fiercely held independence. She deeply resented not being able to gallivant about as she had done, as she was so very used to doing.

The three accounts of Jane's treatment plan that have concluded the final story in this chapter, typify the two most common approaches to medical interpretations of health and illness. These are the naturalistic approach, the familiar territory of clinicians which objectifies biological dysfunction, and the normative approach of the social sciences that evaluates illness in social terms (Carel, 2008). Yet neither of these positions satisfactorily accommodate the sufferer's perspective on what it is to be ill. The philosopher Havi Carel on discovering she had a life-limiting lung condition, decided to investigate the phenomenology of illness. She argues that it is living in the present that can most overcome the suffering of past memories and future fears, and concludes "Sometimes my illness makes life hard. It often takes up more time and space than I would like it to. But it has also given me an ability to be truly happy in the present, in being here and now" (Carel, 2008: 135).

In the next chapter, I believe the evidence described will fully endorses Carel's thesis in relation to Jane's experience of life-limiting illness. This chapter has presented the first three stories: Wondering, Finding, and Planning. Data from all three substantive sources: Jane's blog, my interview recollections, and the health records were used to detail the first few weeks of the Illness Period interspersed with references to the academic literature at salient points.

Notes

1. Blog post 'Home', December 2010.
2. Blog post 'Epiphany', January 2011.
3. This episode was prior to Dr Kate Granger's #hello my name is campaign (http://hellomynameis.org.uk).
4. Here I cannot be precise about when this was – I remember we had a conversation about the music and indeed it was one of her 'things'.

5 By way of a reminder I did not actually see the health records until I was able to access them two years later for this study. We only had sight of the hospital discharge letters at the time.
6 When I had access to the health records I saw the blood was taken but it was never sent for genetic testing as presumably the funding was not forthcoming.
7 www.cancerresearchuk.org/our-research/our-research-by-cancer-subject/our-research-on-clinical-trials
8 This is a year after Jane's death.
9 www.ovacome.org.uk/campaigning-volunteering/beat/
10 By this I mean surgical house officers (SHOs) and recently qualified GPs.

References

Alsop, Christiane Kraft (2002) 'Home and away: self-reflexive auto-ethnography', *Forum: Qualitative Social Research*, 3

Anand, Sumit & Malhi, Gin S (2011) 'From manual to bible: the questionable hegemony of DSM IV', *Australian & New Zealand Journal of Psychiatry*, 45, 5, 348–350

Aujoulat, Isabelle, Luminet, Olivier & Deccache, Alain (2007) 'The perspective of patients on their experience of powerlessness', *Qualitative Health Research*, 17, 6, 772–785

Ayantunde, A A & Parsons, S L (2007) 'Pattern and prognostic factors in patients with malignant ascites: a retrospective study', *Annals of Oncology*, 18, 945–949

Brendtro, Larry K & Mitchell, Martin L (2013) 'The vital balance: becoming weller than well', *Reclaiming Children & Youth*, 22, 2, 5–9

Burke, Brian L, Martens, Andy & Faucher, Erik H (2010) 'Two decades of terror management theory: a meta-analysis of mortality salience research', *Personality & Social Psychology Review*, 14, 155–195

Busfield, Joan (2010) '"A pill for every ill": explaining the expansion in medicine use', *Social Science & Medicine*, 70, 6, 934–941

Butler, Sandra & Rosenblum, Barbara (1991) *Cancer in Two Voices*, San Francisco: Spinsters Ink Books

Campen, Cretien van (2014) *The Proust Effect: The Senses as Doorways to Lost Memories*, Oxford: Oxford University Press

Cannon, Walter (1932) *Wisdom of the Body*, United States: W W Norton & Company

Carel, Havi (2008) *Illness*, Durham: Acumen Publishing

Coutts, Marion (2014) *The Iceberg: A Memoir*, London: Atlantic Books

Farah, Martha J (2002) 'Emerging ethical issues in neuroscience', *Nature Neuroscience*, 5, 11, 1123–1129

Gadamer, Hans-Georg (2004) *Truth and Method*, New York: Continuum International Publishing Group Ltd, 2nd edition

Goldbeck, Rainer (1997) 'Denial in physical illness', *Journal of Psychosomatic Research*, 43, 575–593

Greenberg, J, Pyszczynski, T & Solomon, S (1986) 'The causes and consequences of a need for self-esteem: a terror management theory', in R F Baumeister, Ed., *Public Self and Private Self*, New York: Springer-Verlag

Habbema, J D, Collins, J, Leridon, H, Evers, J L, Lunenfeld, B, & te Velde, E R (2004) 'Towards less confusing terminology in reproductive medicine: a proposal', *Human Reproduction*, 19, 7, 1497–1501

Hagerty, R G, Butow, P N, Ellis, P M, Dimitry, S & Tattersall, M H (2005) 'Communicating prognosis in cancer care: a systematic review of the literature', *Annals of Oncology*, 16, 7, 1005–1053

Hamilton, W (2012) 'Computer assisted diagnosis of ovarian cancer in primary care', *British Medical Journal*, 344: d7628

Hannay, D R (1980) '"The iceberg" of illness and "trivial" consultations', *Journal of the Royal College of General Practitioners*, 30, 551–554

Hermans, Hubert J M (2001) 'The dialogical self: toward a theory of personal and cultural positioning', *Culture & Psychology*, 7, 243–281

Jenkinson, Audrey (2004) *Past Caring*, Clifton-upon-Teme: Polperro Heritage Press

Kirwan, John M J, Tincello, Douglas G, Herod, Jonathan J O, Frost, Olive & Kingston, Robert E (2002) 'Effect of delays in primary care referral on survival of women with epithelial ovarian cancer: retrospective audit', *British Medical Journal*, 324, 7330, 148–151

Lambek, M (2003) 'Introduction: irony and illness – recognition and refusal', *Social Analysis*, 47, 2, 1–19

Last, J M & Adelaide, D P (1963) 'The iceberg: "completing the clinical picture" in general practice', *The Lancet*, 42, 28–31

Latané, Bibb & Darley, John M (1969) 'Bystander "apathy"', *American Scientist*, 57, 2, 244–268

Madison, Greg (2006) 'Existential migration', *Existential Analysis*, 17, 238–260

Marqusee, Mike (2011) 'Having cancer is an education, and this is what I have learned', *The Guardian*, 26 July

McCorkle, Ruth, Pasacreta, Jeannie & Tang, Siew Tzuh (2003) 'The silent killer: psychological issues in ovarian cancer', *Holistic Nursing Practice*, 17, 300–308

Mechanic, David (1961) 'The concept of illness behaviour', *Journal of Chronic Disease*, 15, 189–194

Moynihan, Ray, Doust, Jenny & Henry, David (2012) 'Preventing overdiagnosis: how to stop harming the healthy', *British Medical Journal*, 344, e3502

Murphy, Kathleen (1992) 'The last temptation of Sigourney Weaver', *Film Comment*, 28, 4, 17–20

Newbury, Margaret J (2009) *The Carer's Initiation: A Qualitative Study of the Experience of Family Care of the Dying*, Professional Doctorate in Health thesis, Bath: University of Bath

NICE (2011) *Ovarian Cancer: The Recognition and Initial Management of Ovarian Cancer*, Manchester: National Institute for Health and Clinical Excellence, 122

Plenderleith, Helen Jane (1993) 'An approach to Goethe's treatment of religion in *Dichtung und Wahrheit*', *German Life & Letters*, 46, 297–310

Radley, Alan (2004) 'Recognizing symptoms and falling ill', in *Making Sense of Illness: The Social Psychology of Health and Disease*, London: SAGE Publications Ltd, 61–84

Rayson, Daniel (2013) 'On denying denial', *Journal of Clinical Oncology*, 31, 4371–4372

Rossing, M A, Wicklund, K G, Cushing-Haugen, K L & Weiss, N S (2010) 'Predictive value of symptoms for early detection of ovarian cancer', *Journal of National Cancer Institute*, 102, 4, 222–229

Salander, Pär (2002) 'Bad news from the patient's perspective: an analysis of the written narratives of newly diagnosed cancer patients', *Social Science & Medicine*, 55, 721–732

Sand, Lisa, Strang, Peter & Milberg, Anna (2008) 'Dying cancer patients' experiences of powerlessness and helplessness', *Support Care Cancer*, 16, 7, 853–862

Schaepe, Karen Sue (2011) 'Bad news and first impressions: patient and family caregiver accounts of learning the cancer diagnosis', *Social Science & Medicine*, 73, 6, 912–921

SIGN (2003) *Epithelial Ovarian Cancer*, Edinburgh: Scottish Intercollegiate Guidelines Network, 75

SIGN (2013) *Epithelial Ovarian Cancer*, Edinburgh: Scottish Intercollegiate Guidelines Network, 135

Smith, Lucy K, Pope, Catherine & Botha, Johannes L (2005) 'Patients' help-seeking experiences and delay in cancer presentation: a qualitative synthesis', *The Lancet*, 366, 825–831

SOED (2007) *Shorter Oxford English Dictionary*, Oxford: Oxford University Press

Stacey, Jackie (1997) *Teratologies: A Cultural Study of Cancer*, London: Routledge
Sullivan, Stephen N (2012) 'Functional abdominal bloating with distention', *ISRN Gastroenterology*, 2012, 1–5
Svenaeus, Fredrik (2003) 'Das Unheimliche: towards a phenomenology of illness', *Medicine, Health Care, & Philosophy*, 3, 3–16
Todres, Les (2008) 'Being with that: the relevance of embodied understanding for practice', *Qualitative Health Research*, 18, 1566–73
Todres, Les & Galvin, Kathleen T (2008) 'Embodied interpretation: a novel way of evocatively re-presenting meanings in phenomenological research', *Qualitative Research*, 8, 5, 568–583
Trimble, E L, Ungerleider, R S, Abrams, J A, Kaplan, R S, Feigal, E G, Smith, M A, Carter, C L & Friedman, M A (1993) 'Neoadjuvant therapy in cancer treatment', *CANCER Supplement*, 72, 11
Vos, M S & de Haes, J C J M (2007) 'Denial in cancer patients: an explorative review', *Psycho-Oncology*, 16, 12–25
Wilcock, Ann Allart (1999) 'Reflections on doing, being and becoming', *Australian Occupational Therapy Journal*, 46, 1–11
Zerubavel, E (2006) *The Elephant in the Room: Silence and Denial in Everyday Life*, Oxford: Oxford University Press
Zola, Irving Kenneth (1973) 'Pathways to the doctor: from person to patient', *Social Science & Medicine*, 7, 9, 677–689

3
DAYS FOR DANCING

This chapter covers the longest period in the Dance to Death, a total of 147 days and spans six months. It begins with the pivotal point from the previous chapter when the diagnosis has been confirmed and plans for treatment with chemotherapy have been agreed. Again there are three stories: Treating, Turning and Living. As before, these titles reflect the defining theme during each phase.

Treating

Following the first clinic consultation, I had assumed we would return to Glasgow. Instead we stay in Edinburgh and visit the botanic gardens where Jane is keen to have her picture taken beside the yew trees.[1] We camp for a second night where it is "so good to be staying in the flat despite the inconvenience" (Personal diary, 14 July 2011). We are so buoyed by the instant treatment plan that the basic accommodation seems irrelevant. I had no real experience of chemotherapy regimes and protocols but I understood the basic process. We are both wide-eyed with ignorance and expectation.

VA: We didn't know anyone who'd been for chemo before so we really didn't know what it was going to be like, how it was going to play out. It started at five o'clock in the morning when she had to take a large amount of dexamethasone and have a banana. We hadn't realised that she would then bounce around for the rest of the night. So I didn't get much sleep and she was as high as a kite. The actual starting process was quite long and involved. There are nice recliner chairs to sit in and you can see out, it's quite a light airy place but there was a lot of stuff to go through, to explain about what the treatment would be like, the kinds of things that we had to do. The problem of infection because Jane's immune system would be hammered, what alternative therapies and vitamins and things she could take or not, what might interfere with the actual treatment. This process of things being explained and lots of leaflets and stuff like that took at least an hour, it did just seem to go on for a long time.

Then the actual treatment cycle is quite long, it takes hours because there's a number of different drugs that have to be given to try and prevent nausea and vomiting. The other thing that you become so aware of is that because everybody has one or more infusion pumps, they're constantly beeping. Some of the infusions are only about 15 minutes and then they beep, beep, beep so there's this constant melody. Except it's not really a melody at all, just a cacophony of beeps. It could really get to you but of course the staff develop that way of hearing but not hearing so they're oblivious to it but it's quite strange. There were lots of other people there already whose treatment had started, many of whom had already lost their hair but generally it was quite a calm, relaxed sort of place.

Once Jane had been clerked in and they were going to start the treatment I said I would wait until the first actual chemotherapy agent started. Then I would go off for an hour because it didn't seem appropriate although there wasn't a problem with me staying with Jane. I didn't want to get in the way and so once she'd had her milkshakes and things, I went away for an hour and then came back and treatment was still going. Then more flushings and so on and eventually it was all done. But we'd been there all day and it was quite exhausting. Even things like trying to go to the loo because you've got this drip stand with these pumps. So she would wait until I was there to take her, not because she needed to be taken but it was just a question of manoeuvring things and opening doors and then it was easier if I was standing outside so she didn't have to worry about locking the door.

INTERVIEWER: What I'm hearing is that you got a very different feel of this place than you had of the consultation the day before, there wasn't a tension here.

VA: Yes, that's right. Although the place was very busy, I suppose it reminded me a bit of A & E, that bustle of efficiency. The patients were in recliner chairs and it was calm, it wasn't anything like as bad as I had thought it was going to be.

(Interview Three, 20 August 2013)

Reflecting on the episode now, both my interview recollection and the memories that foregrounds, it occurs to me that the rapidity with which treatment was started was the most considerate event in the whole saga. There was no time to worry or further anticipate what might happen. Overnight the gloom of the formal diagnosis was quashed by the quick start of the treatment. At the time we were just impressed by the efforts of the oncologist. It is clear however, from the surgeon's notes of the first Gynaecology Cancer Multidisciplinary Meeting (MDM), that the team were moved by Jane's plight. Under the heading *Clinical details* is the cryptic phrase "3C ovarian min, dreadful burden, neo A +/- primary" (MDM hospital record, day 30). Otherwise the form is simply a hospital note that accounts for a discussion about a particular patient, their disease and the treatment plan. The detail of who was present and what was discussed is not recorded. Mattingly (1998) distinguishes between the recorded 'chart talk' of clinical detail which emphasises pathology and diagnosis and the discussion of patients' personal stories which have "no formal status as a vehicle for clinical reasoning" (Mattingly, 1998: 273). The awfulness of this particular woman's situation and its reality is encapsulated by the expression 'dreadful burden'. It may seem unnecessary to ask who had the burden? It was most probably intended to refer to the burden being carried by a woman with an advanced gynaecological cancer but the term burden has other, quantifiable meanings in health care.

In 1990, the World Health Organization (WHO) and the World Bank commissioned the Harvard School of Public Health to quantify death numbers worldwide and to take into account the impact of disease and disability on populations. The research was reported as the Global Burden of Disease Study.[2] The result was a single measurement termed the overall "burden of disease" (Murray & Lopez, 1996: 2). The study team used time as a common currency to determine the impact of disease or disability on what might have otherwise been expected in a healthy lifespan. Two key standardised measures were devised: the Quality-Adjusted Life Year (QALY) and the Disability-Adjusted Life Year (DALY). The quantification of health care interventions in terms of cost effectiveness was not new, especially not in the USA where such services are not free at the point of delivery. The post-war interest in affluence and the subsequent attention to human relations in the 1960s, have been attributed as key factors to the rise of health economics (Robinson, 1986). The related term, Quality of Life (QoL) is described as 'ubiquitous' (Fallowfield, 2009: 1) because it can be measured and defined in so many ways, making comparisons difficult. Nevertheless, in a systematic review it was found to be a helpful measure for improving survival outcomes in cancer patients when used as a prognostic indicator prior to treatment (Montazeri, 2009). The clinical team with responsibility for Jane's treatment plan were also familiar with the concept through their local guidelines:

> Treatment is not usually curative. ... The goal for healthcare professionals must be to ensure that where cure is not possible a woman can have a good quality of life with judicious use of surgery and chemotherapy.
>
> (SIGN, 2013: 1)

This seems to confirm the judicious nature of the treatment plan which was to try the chemotherapy protocol but it was known and accepted that even this was unlikely to be successful and that cure was impossible. Miracles were not discussed.

There are other ways of exploring the concept of burden in relation to the study which go beyond health economics. At this point in the narrative, the burden of the disease for Jane and for me as her partner and carer, had not fully emerged. As I wrote that last sentence, I was conscious of typing *partner* before *carer* because that came first in our relationship, but I now realise the roles switched as I became *carer* first and *partner* second. The burden that we were aware of at this time was the physical weight and girth of Jane's abdomen. Perhaps there was also the burden that was shared by all who were directly involved in Jane's care, the multi-disciplinary team, that is the emotional burden of the knowledge of the extent of her disease. It may be helpful to distinguish between the personal burden for the individual as the disease affects the physical, psychological, social and financial aspects of daily life, and the global burden as outlined above. However, this falls into the trap of reifying illness as a medico-scientific commodity which would then allow someone to distance themselves from the disease by claiming they are a victim of external forces (Bury, 1982). Viewed in this way, the ill person does not need "to accept fully the burden of responsibility" (Bury, 1982: 173). As a result of improving health care and the decline of infectious diseases, chronic illness is an increasing burden for health care systems and providers. More recently, the burden of treatment has been recognised as a feature of chronic illness:

> patients experience new and growing demands to organise and co-ordinate their own care, to comply with complex treatment and self-monitoring regimens, and to meet a whole range of expectations of personal motivation, expertise and self-care.
>
> (May et al., 2014: 2)

The authors go on to propose a model designed to capitalise on the patient's social networks in the pursuit and support of patient-centred care. Earlier, I noted that the dance had begun with the formation of Jane's social network, the basis of her support. Now, as we come to understand the burden of the treatment regime, so the complexity of the dance is realised. Jane summarises the first chemotherapy session and what would become a typical chemo day:

> Chemotherapy is a fascinating process. I think perhaps some people are scared of it, because it's poison, and because it makes your hair fall out. But it's the medicine, it gets rid of the cancer, it's what makes you better. The dialectic of toxicity, kill/cure, creation/destruction, is quite hard to get your head around. Remember when we were in Belgium in February and Parsifal had such an effect on us? One of the key themes is the healing power of poison, but we never thought at the time that this would strike home with quite such force. My drugs of choice is TaxolCarboplatin based on yew (taxus) and platinum. The day before the first session [we went] to the Botanics to commune with the yew trees (and maybe we'll get those platinum eternity rings after all…)
>
> The chemo cycle starts in the middle of the night before when I have to take a massive dose of steroids (which make me rather bouncy, some might say aggressive although only towards my pillows, but are intended to prevent nausea). I reported to [the chemotherapy ward] and a lovely young nurse sat with us for over an hour explaining the procedures, possible side effects, risks (the big one is infection), whom to contact with any queries (24 hour cover, no question or concern too trivial) and my forward treatment plan.

> Then I sat in a reclining chair by an open window above a flower garden from around 11 until shortly before 5 while various fluids coursed through my veins (the yew and the platinum, interspersed with saline, antihistamines, steroids and various other things to counteract side-effects). It was a really interesting day, for the procedure itself, for the people also undergoing treatment, for the calm, kind, incredibly busy efficiency of the nurses.
>
> *(Blog post 'Silver Linings', 28 July 2011)*

The first paragraph introduces two important features of Jane's personal philosophy and my interpretation of the path to the aesthetic experience of dying. I do not propose to discuss the latter point at this stage as there is a detailed exploration in Chapter 5. What is noteworthy here is the use of opposites or polarities, and the relevance of symbols. Jane recalls our visit, when we were in Belgium, to a modern production of Wagner's opera *Parsifal*. She wrote a blog post at the time (six months before we knew of her illness) in which she recalls our first (and only) visit to the opera together.

> There was no spear, no chalice, no cross in this production – so quite challenging to follow the plot with the central symbolism absent. There was a lot of veiling, hiding and camouflage, boundaries and bounds, sexual interplay and duality, ambivalence in the dichotomy of good and evil. The eternal feminine was starkly, barely and intimately central (das Ewigweibliche zieht uns hinan).
>
> *(Blog post 'A Night at the Opera', 26 January 2011)*

Her quotation is from the closing lines of *Faust* translated as "Eternal womanhood draws us all on" (Goethe, 2007: 372). Conventionally this is interpreted as Faust's salvation but Jantz (1953) finds a deeper, more potent meaning that I doubt was lost on Jane. He argues that the entire play centres on the realisation of the symbolic essence of truth through the principle of what he translates as 'the eternal womanly' and defines as "the feminine principle of love, of mercy and grace, which leads the spirit upward to the highest perfection" (Jantz, 1953: 792). Clearly, there is no certainty that in recalling her memories of *Parsifal*, Jane remembers her earlier insights. I suspect she does and draws strength as Gadamer (2004) suggests through an inner fusion of her understanding (of Goethe) and interpretation with the practical application of an actual text, that is *Faust*. She may well have reached a realisation similar to that proposed by Jantz:

> The 'Eternal-Womanly', therefore, was unmistakably intended by Goethe to comprise in symbolic form the great creative continuity of life, birth and rebirth in constantly renewed forms, the ultimate resolution of death, destruction, and tragedy in new cycles of life, constructive activity, and fulfilment.
>
> *(Jantz, 1953: para 804)*

It is likely that she drew upon this interpretation in her understanding of one of the Parsifal themes, that of a healing poison. This is the Paracelsian notion that it is the dose that makes the poison or "the thing that harms is also the thing that heals" (Jung, 1971: para 373). In the blog excerpt two polarities are identified: kill – cure and creation – destruction. Both are highly relevant to someone undergoing a toxic treatment to *kill* by *destruction* that which the body has *created* although the possibility of *cure* was understood to be remote. The use of polarities was recognised by Jung in his interpretation of the Parsifal story:

> Under the spell of Klingsor is Kundry, symbolising the instinctive life-force or libido that Amfortas lacks. Parsifal ... free from opposites, is therefore the redeemer, the bestower of healing and renewed vitality, who unites the bright, heavenly, feminine symbol of the Grail with the dark, earthly, masculine symbol of the spear.
>
> *(Jung, 1971: para 371)*

It is also worth noting the central themes of Wagner's last opera which reveal a deeper parallel: suffering, pain, compassion and redemption (Kinderman & Syer, 2005).

Returning to the story, treatment has started and many adjustments are needed to the step sequence of our lives as we learn to accommodate the practical implications of chemotherapy. We return to Glasgow following the first session where Jane's mother and our cats have to be indoctrinated in the new hygiene regime:

INTERVIEWER: Okay, you say that we're getting our heads round the various drugs and behaviours [referring to storyboard], and I'm wondering what behaviours?

VA: Well we're now back through in Glasgow and so her body has been hammered by these highly toxic agents and we've got to be really careful about infection. So we were both pretty good at hand-washing anyway but hand-washing has been taken to new heights. But it's not as simple as just the two of us, it involves her mum as well and that was quite difficult and we were on tenter-hooks that Jane would then catch something. We also had the cats and the cat litter and didn't want the cats bouncing around with stuff. There were also drugs to take because the anti-emetics have to continue for a few days after and there was also tailing off of the steroids as well.

INTERVIEWER: How did Jane get her head round this?

VA: Well she didn't really have to do too much because I just took over and instigated whatever hygiene arrangements needed to be done. What she did was to make sure that she washed her hands and she would avoid going too close to people. She knew that she had to be careful about going up and hugging people, not to directly kiss people and so on. Also to be careful with the cats and that if she did go outside or if she touched anything. But there were even things like she had to be careful if she touched house plants because of course she would then excrete through her skin.

(Interview Three, 20 August 2013)

This extract illustrates the additional difficulties we both faced by not being, or feeling, 'at home' and the added anxiety of the effect the illness was having on others. Jane wants to protect her mother who is disempowered by my presence in the primary caring role. Feeling relaxed has become impossible even when asleep in the uncomfortable bed arrangements although this is soon remedied by having a duvet underneath. The parallel activities of making our new home habitable continue but plans to decorate the entire flat ourselves are abandoned in favour of professional decorators. We decide to stay in a guesthouse for a few nights of relative comfort and to supervise flat improvements. My brother and his partner visit at this time and stay with friends nearby. I email my sister with a progress report:

> Hi – We had a grand week (4 nights) in Portobello and it was great to see [my brother and his partner]. The guest house we stayed in was very accommodating of her majesty's special requirements including not coming in to 'clean' the room, allowing access at all times and generally being kind and understanding. So far the chemo has been fine – Jane has been quite tired on occasion and the swollen belly hasn't helped but the new GP has prescribed posh oil of peppermint capsules and it now seems to be improving, also the protein drinks are helping with the water-logging. And we're home alone this weekend which suits very well. It's not been so easy in recent weeks as [Jane's mother's] doesn't really get the germ paranoia and has a tendency to sneezing fits within royal airspace. I have some inkling of what motherhood might have been like as I manoeuvre her majesty past obstacles, fending off small children and sneezers, while swabbing surfaces with an ever-present packet of hand wipes from my satchel.
> *(Personal email, 30 July 2011)*

The timing of my brother's visit was fortuitous, originally arranged to visit our demented mother in her care home but now Jane and I both need to feel and draw upon the strength of (my) family. However, the treatment regime and its necessary behaviours are compounding an already difficult situation.

INTERVIEWER: And at this stage you're saying a bit about the family reacting strangely at times and mostly staying away.

VA: Well the message had gone out on the jungle drums that infection control was in place and that if they had a cold or anything like that they [her family] were to stay, well they weren't to stay away but they were to keep their distance. Her mum certainly went out quite a lot and it was really difficult for her because this was an awful thing that was happening to her daughter and it was hard to watch.

INTERVIEWER: How did Jane react to them not really knowing what to do and staying away, that bit of tension around that?

VA: She found that quite hard because it was about finding a balance between understanding that somebody's at risk of infection and there are some simple measures that need to happen but that doesn't mean to say that people can't visit. I think because I was guarding Jane to such an extent that was possibly part of it as well. There was a slight feeling that the infection control was a good excuse, it made it easier for people who would have found it difficult to visit, to say oh well I've got a bit of a snuffle.

(Interview Three, 20 August 2013)

It was a very difficult time for everyone and the repercussions within a family take time to settle. Where studies have been done these tend to focus on spousal response (see for example Wilson & Morse, 1991 and Hilton et al., 2000) or on family survival (Mellon & Northouse, 2001). This was perhaps simply part of an adjustment process where family members reflected on their positions in response to the shocking news. The treatment process is affecting Jane:

VA: There was an overwhelming weariness, she wasn't sleeping particularly well, she wasn't comfortable in bed. Then all of this stuff had happened to her in a quite short space of time. She'd just completely been through the wringer, she needed to gather herself together. I suppose we had gone into the excitement of the treatment phase buoyed up not only by the apparent positiveness of the oncologist but also with the amount of steroids that she was given. Actually we were just charging up a cliff and we'd both jumped off and she now needed to deal with the consequences as we hit the ground quite hard.

INTERVIEWER: So was this a time of hitting the ground quite hard?

VA: Yes, I think so. I'm not very, I was going to say I'm not very patient. In some situations I can be very patient but I generally tend to be impatient for things to happen and so, yes we knew what this was, yes we knew what the treatment was now she can be better. But it wasn't going to be like that and she wasn't going to be instantly better in fact I knew she wasn't going to be better at all.

INTERVIEWER: So were you the one who hit the ground quite hard at this time?

VA: No, I kept moving. I felt it was really important that I was very positive. We'd had the tears and the angst following the diagnosis but I tried very hard to keep it together for Jane. It was hard enough for her without me crumbling, so I just kept busy.

(Interview Three, 20 August 2013)

And it is not just the tiredness from the treatment that is having an effect. We both knew her hair would fall out, warned by the oncologist, but neither of us are ready for the real impact:

INTERVIEWER: And how did she respond to her hair coming out?

VA: I think within three weeks of her having the chemo, it started to come out. That was awful, that was really hard for her, she knew it would come out. There was clumps of it on the pillow and stuff in bed and it's one thing knowing it's going to happen, it's quite another thing watching it happen. So

I cut it short but then within a few days it was getting really patchy and it looked a mess so I said maybe we just need to bite the bullet and get rid of the whole thing so that you've got a nice smooth pate. Her father had gone bald and so that was okay. I was very conscious of that person, of how she looked then, had gone. Her hair would never grow in the same again, she would never look like that again. She'd had beautifully thick hair, but that was it, gone.

INTERVIEWER: And I'm hearing how significant that was for you that sense that it would never come back the same. How was it for her do you think?

VA: I think it was one of the hardest parts of the chemo, in fact, it was probably the hardest part. It was one thing being hammered by the drugs and feeling tired and like you had flu and being washed out but the most unpleasant side-effect was losing her hair and it wasn't quite a Samson and Delilah loss of strength. She didn't want a wig, she didn't want to hide the fact that was what was happening and that's what had happened to her but that's not the same as the effect of actually having had it happen. We're as a society, we're really bad for looking at people and judging them in a particular way and there's a huge sexism in that it's quite chic for men to be bald and complete opposite for women. She felt very disfigured by the loss of her hair.

(Interview Three, 20 August 2013)

Despite being forewarned, the impact of chemotherapy-induced alopecia remains an unfilled challenge in clinical oncology (Roe, 2011; Paus et al., 2013). In a study of women with ovarian cancer, alopecia was seen to be an additional challenge following major gynaecological surgery and a further reminder of a likely early death (Jayde et al., 2013). Accepting changes to bodily appearance has been termed "embodying identity" (Koszalinski & Williams, 2012: 116) to account for the transition the individual must make from self denial to incorporation of the new physical self. Jane however, appears to take hair loss in her stride "We've cut my hair short in anticipation of things to come – it needed cutting, and felt a bit more in control of things to shorten it ourselves" (Blog post 'Portobello', day 47). She continues her positive narrative with tales of future plans for life in Edinburgh:

> We took [my brother and his partner] to the Royal Botanic Garden Edinburgh and showed them all our favourite trees. There's something particularly special about showing a special place to someone else and appreciating their appreciation. By the way I have been accepted onto the Practical Horticulture course starting [in two months time]. My circumstances have changed a bit since application but I'm still hopeful of being able to do it. We went to Ikea and Dobbies, on lighting and garden furniture missions (with lunch). I struggled a bit with crowds, heat and being on my feet at some length but it was worth it to be doing normal things.

(Blog post 'Portobello', 31 July 2011)

Three weeks later she has apparently adjusted to her new appearance and celebrates by publishing her hat design:

> This summer's must-have fashion accessory is the chemo bunnet™. An exclusive range of limited edition headwear has been designed and created by Plenderleith Fashion House of Edinburgh. Handcrafted from delicate, soft bamboo and cotton blends, the chemo bunnet™ is sensitively coloured to grace the bald pate with poise and comfort for any situation inside and outside the home. It's worn just above the ears, eschewing the Benny from Crossroads look, and covers the whole head thus avoiding any potential confusion with the kippah.
>
> *(Blog post 'Essential Accessorising', 19 August 2011)*

Jane has re-invented herself as the woman not just coping with advanced cancer but, with a little self-deprecation, embracing the effects of the treatment on her body by playing with her appearance. This is the public image which she wants to convey to family, friends and anyone else who happens upon the blog; she has a tendency to use it to fend off enquiries from concerned colleagues. In private she does not say how she feels about her alopecia but I know not to ask. When her eyelashes and eyebrows go, she becomes upset and hates the bathroom mirror. Neither of us are good with make-up and although an attempt is made with eye-liner and eye-brow pencil, she looks like a clown. Efforts are promptly abandoned in favour of hair-free honesty, a reaction similar to the suggestion that some women react through provocation when "baldness is seen as the symbol of the cancer patient's new identity" (Rosman, 2004: 333).

By day 50, we have decided to move into the now painted and carpeted flat, and live through the disruption of the kitchen installation. Over the next fortnight, possessions and cats are brought from Glasgow, and the furniture arrives from storage in the Highlands. To avoid the trip hazards of unnecessary clutter, much of our belongings go straight back into storage but now it is at least nearby. Jane was not alone with the breezy public face as illustrated by email correspondence with my sister:

> Hi – I don't know if you & Jane had thought more about us coming over or not but we think it might be better just to wait until Christmas. Obviously it will mean waiting longer to see you which is a shame but I think, under the circumstances, it might be as well not to have the prospect of visitors at a time when you will both have more important things to attend to. Talk to you about all this and more soon. Thought I might phone on Saturday. Very much love to you and our dear Queen.
>
> *(Personal email from my sister, 3 August 2011)*

> Hi – Here we are in [the flat] after quite a busy day of hoovering and grout scrubbing royale. You may well be right about waiting until Christmas

although I still think it's worth booking the flights as they'll only go up. We now know there are 4 chemo cycles and a CT scan before a review [in three weeks]. Hopefully the knives will then be sharpened and that will take a few weeks to get over. We can speak about on Saturday – all telecoms functioning well so phone or Skype is fine. Eyes are starting to cross so I'd better stop this and put the light out.

Speak soon, much love from me and the hairless queen

(Personal email to my sister, 3 August 2011)

It would be a gross understatement to say that I had not thought about my sister visiting from Canada where she lives; it was one of my first thoughts when I realised the severity of Jane's illness. But I also knew that disrupting her life was unfair, that she would come in an instant if I asked yet it was a visit that needed to be timed to perfection. That moment that would come when Jane was well enough to enjoy the visit although she might not live much longer. So a family Christmas in three months' time seemed an ideal opportunity for everyone to be together albeit as I knew, for one last time. How I knew was based on my previous nursing experience and the advanced state of the disease. Later I was able to predict with some accuracy (a very dark art) Jane's likely demise based on her tumour marker levels.

So around day 50 we were both playing a game of 'keeping up appearances' and using humour to keep everyone's mood light. At the end of a blog post on the practicalities of living with minimal equipment and furniture, Jane describes her glabrous state:

> I'm now magnificently bald, by the way, although some grey fuzz has started to reappear which looks and feels a bit odd. A bit self-conscious, I've been alert to people's reactions – some give me a big broad smile, some look away, most don't seem to notice. Being bald is only a stigma for women, of course. But as [my sister] says, rumour has it I'm too sexy for my hair.
>
> *(Blog post 'Indoor Camping', 15 August 2011)*

What Jane does not write about is the correspondence she has with her cousin's daughter who was studying biochemistry. It starts innocently following the email she sent to everyone regarding our change of address but soon becomes a frank discussion:

COUSIN: I did a module in cancer biology last semester. How much do you know about what you've got?

JANE: I have a Stage 3 serous tumour which started on my left ovary (or fallopian tube, there is apparently some debate), has munched through most of my uterus and 'involves' the bladder and the rectum. I've learned a little about BRCA1 and BRCA2[3] mutations but mostly just from wikipedia. [The oncologist's] taken some blood for DNA analysis if he can include me in his study. Somehow making a contribution to research makes me feel a whole lot better. That much I know. I'd really like to chat to you about this, objectifying the condition also helps me to deal with it.

COUSIN: I didn't realise BRCA1 and BRCA2 were related to ovarian cancer – I don't know an awful lot about them, except that BRCA2 is the most common genetic cause of male breast cancer, and that they're involved in DNA repair – as most oncogenes are.

I found your blog entry, very interesting read – I'm glad the NHS is taking care of you, and the lovely oncologist does sound lovely. It's also great that you've been able (hopefully) to contribute to his research; I suppose as an academic it's sort of built in, in a way, isn't it? Objectifying I can absolutely do, and it's been forever since we last actually spoke so it'd be great to catch up.

Are you bald already? (she asked, tactfully...) I'm not sure how quickly the chemo will knock out your follicles. I'm sure it can't be fun, having your hair fall out, but it does mean the chemo's working – the drugs target rapidly dividing cells, because that's what your tumour is doing, but it's also what your hair, and the lining of your gut, is doing.

(Personal email, 8–12 August 2011)

This exchange is followed by a lengthy discussion on the finer points of oncogenes and genetic mutations. I am deliberately out at the time but Jane says it was helpful and good to catch up. I do remember that she was immensely impressed by her scientific cousin's knowledge and the intellectual quality of the discussion. This young woman was able to provide credible, scientific information early in Jane's illness and treatment when others either mollified (the gynaecological cancer clinical nurse specialist) or just did not know (much of this was new to me). I feel relieved she is talking to someone about her condition although not perhaps her situation. We continue our dance, still trying to master the steps but getting the rhythm:

>Week before treatment visit GP for chemo bloods > Chemo session > Week after feel a bit grim > Next week feel better > Week before treatment visit GP for chemo bloods

Then a variation, a letter arrives instructing Jane to attend for a CT scan of her abdomen. The appointment will take an hour which seems a long time for a scan but the reason soon becomes clear:

A nurse came out and said that Jane had to drink this contrast medium which was a litre jug. Jane found large volumes of things quite difficult and she had to drink it within an hour. So she started to try and drink but she was getting overwhelmed by this volume of stuff. We had to work quite hard at keeping her calm, reassuring her that no she wasn't going to throw up. She really did struggle with drinking it all and there was a lot of clock-watching. Eventually she managed to drink all the stuff and went off for the scan.

(Interview Four, 27 August 2013)

We are not warned that Jane needs to drink the litre of fluid prior to the scan but then I doubt if the staff can empathise with feeling full to the brim and then being asked to drink a litre, in forty minutes. It seems a cruel irony that in order to evaluate the progress of the treatment, another torture has to be endured. Jane stoically understands the need for the scan and the discomfort but it is a hard experience for us both. The result of the scan is reported within a few days, before the clinic appointment the following week, but the oncologist telephones on the day Jane has been for her usual blood tests. He is concerned that the spreading disease is in danger of affecting Jane's right kidney, the one that continues to function. My trump card, which saves Jane from an interim hospital visit, is the blood tests from earlier that afternoon. The oncologist is able to check the results and confirm that despite the scan report, Jane's kidney function is fine.

However, the clinic visit the following week was rather tense as I recall. It may seem trite to say that Jane wanted a good report but the actual meeting was difficult:

> The oncologist broke the news, not particularly gently I felt, that the CT scan after the third chemo cycle showed that the tumour had not apparently shrunk very much. Certainly not enough for them to consider surgery at this stage. He asked if this news surprised me. I think I nodded, while actually it would be more accurate to say that it rather floored me. Because I had been feeling so much better, and stronger (and smaller, the swelling having reduced significantly), I was sure the chemo was working and that surgery would be scheduled soon. Instead [the oncologist] has proposed a new weekly chemo regime, which means a bit less of the chemicals at one go, but more often. For the next few months our weekly plans will have to be organised around blood tests and hospital days. As the doctor in the cancer unit put it, it's changing from a bazooka-type approach to a machine gun.
>
> (Blog post, 'A Different Mindset', 20 September 2011)

The report of the MDM meeting prior to the clinic session, affords another explanation for the oncologist's apparent abruptness:

> This lady's case was discussed at the Combined Gynae Oncology Meeting and I saw at the clinic thereafter. As you know she has now received 3 cycles of three weekly Carboplatin and Paclitaxel chemotherapy for a grade 3 stage 3C serous papillary ovarian carcinoma. Previous laparoscopy had shown the disease to be extremely extensive and certainly inoperable at that point. Unfortunately the lady's CA-125 level has gradually crept up on chemotherapy having been 8967 at the start rising to 9184 after 2 cycles. In terms of a percent change this is clearly minimal. Radiology from pre-chemotherapy compared to post-chemotherapy suggested the disease has remained largely stable but that there is worsening hydronephrosis. Discussion at the Multidisciplinary Team

revolved around the fact that this lady appeared to have very resistant disease and that we should change her to weekly Carboplatin and Paclitaxel.

(Hospital record, 8 September 2011)

This was probably not the discussion that the team wanted to have but they were also aware that a good response to the chemotherapy was unlikely. Not only did the scan show a worsening of the disease, the CA-125 tumour marker was rising not falling. While Catt et al. (2005) have reported that MDMs can be beneficial for both patients and health professionals, the emotional strain on the team, particularly its leaders (the oncologist and the surgeon) can also be an issue for some. Others have suggested that clinicians with high job satisfaction through status and research (Ramirez, 1996) develop a range of coping strategies to offset the stresses and strains of their jobs (Bates, 1982). However, there will always be difficult cases such as those affecting younger people who often present with advanced and therefore untreatable disease. The team had previously discussed the 'dreadful burden' of this particular case and now, despite three cycles of chemotherapy, the scan and tumour marker results indicated disease progression with no sign of remission. The oncologist's irritation can perhaps be understood as frustration at the impotence of the treatment and the likely impossibility of remission (Stiefel & Krenz, 2013). The oncologist's version of the encounter suggests a more positive mood:

When I actually saw the lady at the clinic she told me that symptomatically she felt much better since starting the chemotherapy with more energy and resolution of her abdominal pain. She admits some abdominal distension still persists. In terms of toxicity to chemotherapy the only major side effect has been alopecia. Fatigue was an issue after cycle 1 but this has decreased as time went on.

(MDM hospital record, 8 September 2011)

In those first few weeks following the diagnosis, it was easy to be carried along with the rapid response by the health professionals to start treatment. Equally, as we learnt the new dance to our hope of remission, it was easy to push away the dark thoughts of reality. Now a much more vigorous dance is needed but I want Jane to start directing it, to make the decisions herself:

INTERVIEWER: So you said that after the phone call that you were brought up sharp about the seriousness of it and this was the same seriousness really getting emphasised here?
VA: Yes.
INTERVIEWER: And how did Jane respond to that?
VA: She was quiet, she didn't. But there was still something to do, there was a modified plan so okay, plan A hasn't worked but we've got plan B here so we'll start with that. So the aggressive tumour is met with more aggressive treatment so they're having a good fight for her.
INTERVIEWER: So they're fighting for her?

VA: Yes.

INTERVIEWER: And is that, would that be how Jane understood what was happening do you think?

VA: Yes, that they were putting up their best efforts, they were really trying to sort this so there was still a veneer of optimism?

INTERVIEWER: A veneer?

VA: Yes.

INTERVIEWER: And I'm sort of hearing that you and she perhaps didn't really go below the veneer.

VA: I had started to feel, I had been feeling that she was detaching herself from the body that had gone wrong, that need to be treated, and herself. She had to take responsibility for what might happen to her and she needed to be in control of what was done. There would inevitably be some very difficult choices. I knew what the surgery would involve, that we weren't just talking about going in and taking out the bad bit, they would take out quite a lot of other bits as well which would result in colostomies and all sorts of re-plumbing. The severity of the disease meant that she really did have choices about how much treatment she wanted. But she had to be the one to say.

(Interview Four, 27 August 2013)

In this exchange, I seem to be struggling with what to say in response to the interviewer's questions and prompts. I am floundering as I remember not saying what I knew about Jane's condition. I want her to know how bad it is, to face reality but I sense she is not yet ready. Despite the difficult news, it is only a few days before we are back out enjoying life. Jane is feeling more energetic and enthusiastic than she has for some time. We indulge ourselves in the festival city of culture with visits to the theatre, the military tattoo (sentimental Scot that she was!), art exhibitions and regular excursions to the botanic gardens. She is clambering up nearby hills, revelling in her ability:

> This morning we climbed to the top of Allermuir Hill, the focal point of our living room view. Only 1619 feet high but all achievements are relative and I was very pleased to make it to the top and back down again, feeling stronger and more like myself with every step.
>
> *(Blog post, 'Top of the View', 11 September 2011)*

This particular walk is only three days after the clinic appointment and the realisation that the treatment regime needs to be more aggressive. Jane's response is to climb a mountain both physical and psychological, to get out into the world, to rise above the city and draw strength from a wider landscape.

Turning

The story continues with the adjustments to daily life and the new treatment regime. Following the review at the clinic I have been trying to persuade Jane that she needs to talk to someone about her situation. She has been clear from the outset that she does not want any psychological help despite offers from support services such as the Maggie's Centre. Eventually she concedes to visit a medical herbalist, a meeting that proves to be significant in many ways as I recall:

> [The herbalist] spent a long time talking to Jane. I stayed with Jane but Jane did all the talking and talked about what had happened and the treatment that she was getting and so on. [The herbalist] talked quite a lot about other ways that they were starting to treat certain cancers in other parts of the world like in the US where they actively use herbal therapies alongside cytotoxic agents. We talked about the diet and the difficulty Jane was having with the protein drinks that she was having to take but they were very, very sweet and synthetic tasting, she really hated them. [The herbalist] explained that there were other forms of protein that we could get, powders that were mixed up as a kind of milk shake but nothing like as sweet and more kind of natural tasting. That was really helpful and she would make up some herbal tinctures. The one for Jane had all sorts of things in that were going to support the various things that Jane was feeling and she prescribed other herbs and things too that were thought to help shrink tumours.
>
> But during the conversation Jane suddenly burst into tears and I think it was at that point the enormity of what was going on really hit her. Because somebody was spending much longer talking to her and they were talking to her about her life not just her tumour and her treatment. It was about her and how she lived and what we ate and what we did and that was very different. So we all got a bit upset and then we all got a bit calmer and [the herbalist] advised that Jane perhaps needed to think about doing something to find a calmer place for herself. As she faced each of these challenges of chemo or scans or all the various things that were either being done or potentially might be done to her that she needed some additional tools in her armoury that she didn't currently have. The herbalist has other practitioners there including a counsellor who could teach Jane a visualisation technique. Jane was absolutely adamant that she didn't want to see a counsellor, that she didn't need to talk about the fact that she had cancer, she didn't want to be counselled but she was prepared to go and hear how she could learn and how she could find a calm place for herself.
>
> *(Interview Four, 27 August 2013)*

After the visit I have noted "Yesterday was quite cathartic and we have turned a big corner. J has shifted from passive recipient of treatment to actively trying to shift Tallulah" (Personal diary, day 92). Yet a week passes before Jane describes the visit:

> I've come to realise that chemotherapy is a rather blunt instrument. This realisation has led me to explore other ways of fighting this cancer besides the accepted medical model. I'd set a lot of store by [the oncologist] and the team

doing that 'really good job with the chemo' they needed to do in preparation for surgery. I'd channelled a lot of my energy into believing that this was going to work, and to expressing my confidence in the oncology team as I projected an image of confidence and optimism to family, friends and myself too. This confidence has been a bit shaken, but sometimes a good shake is just what's needed. The wind in the trees shakes out the old, broken branches and dead leaves and lets in the light to the vital, growing stuff at the centre.

I had a bit of an epiphany during the consultation with the herbalist. Actually it was a bit of a crack-up, or a breakdown. At any rate I started to cry, and once I'd started I had some difficulty stopping. I hadn't really had a good cry about the cancer, and as everybody (the herbalist, the nurse in the chemo ward for example) keeps telling me, these emotions are better out than in. Putting my energy into projecting a confident, optimistic front while keeping a lid on my frustrations and fears does not help my body to deal with the cancer. Some people think it's keeping a lid on things that causes cancer in the first place (oncologists think otherwise of course). At any rate I did feel the better of a good cry, and of being able (when I could speak again) to articulate my fears and frustrations. I was upset at myself for not responding as well as was hoped to the chemo. Like not doing as well as I think I should have at my chemo exam and somehow letting myself, and others, down. Old, engrained habits die hard.

(Blog post, 'A Different Mindset', 20 September 2011)

Ten weeks after diagnosis, Jane has now taken ownership of her diagnosis and recognises she has been relying on the health care team to do 'the really good job with the chemo' while she passively complied with treatment and all its necessary intrusions. By looking out and into the new and interesting world of hospital-based therapy, Jane ignored her inner demons appearing to accept her diagnosis and be engaged with its treatment. Her behaviour was neither atypical for her or for others faced with similar situations. Jane tended to 'keep a calm sooch' while suppressing what she felt were undesirable feelings of strong emotion whether they be anger or distress. Laughter, self-deprecation, a comic turn and unadulterated wit she could do with ease but please do not make her cry. Perhaps a rather different mechanism was in play: post-traumatic stress disorder (PTSD) and defined in simple terms as

> a response, sometimes delayed, to an overwhelming event or events, which takes the form of repeated, intrusive hallucinations, dreams or thoughts or behaviours stemming from the event, along with the numbing that may have begun during or after the experience.
>
> *(Caruth, 1995: 4)*

It is not the event itself that results in the response but the failure to assimilate the experience at the time that causes the disorder. A study of women with ovarian cancer found that while overall there was no real difference in the occurrence of PTSD than within the general population, there was an important emergent factor of an avoidant and disengaged coping style (Shand et al., 2014). This was associated with symptoms of PTSD such as substance abuse, self-blame and denial. For Jane substance abuse is not an issue but self-blame and denial are:

> Recognising that it's not my fault is a big thing. Most cancer sufferers apparently think it is their fault, that the tumour is payback time for something they've done (smoked, eaten) in the past. Apparently too there is a strong correlation between introspective, self-critical personalities and cancer (again, this is not a correlation that oncologists would research or recognise).
>
> (Blog post, 'A Different Mindset', 20 September 2011)

In truth, it was perhaps more of a delayed reaction than actual PTSD that Jane felt. Stacey suggests that remembering the traumatic experience, as in the shock of an advanced cancer diagnosis is "a route out of, not into, the experience. The survivor might thus move on from the trauma through a witnessing of the event, rather than a return to it" (Stacey, 1997: 16).

By recalling the experience of the diagnosis in the interview with the herbalist, Jane is able to reflect on it and accept its reality. Jane would have interpreted this as a *return enhanced*, as the interplay between acceptance and rejection. She is able to accept her diagnosis and prognosis when she returns to thinking about it as she recalls the discussion with the herbalist. Previously, she was able to reject the reality of her situation because others were dealing with it for her and taking responsibility. At first glance, it appears she has no choice but to accept the treatment plan. I feel she does have choices, however stark they might be: to have treatment, or not and to explore the alternatives.

In the diary extract above I noted that Jane is actively trying to shift Tallulah and this reference to the tumour by name was noticed by the interviewer who departed from the storyboard script to probe the point:

INTERVIEWER: Okay the thing is the language and the giving of names to so we've had Tigger pills and we've had Tallulah.

VA: Oh well the Tigger pills are the dexamethasone because they just make you bounce and bounce and bounce and even though you haven't really got either the strength or physically able to bounce, you still bounce. I'd forgotten about Tallulah, she'd called the wretched tumour Tallulah but then there was whole thing about Dennis Potter and whether he'd given his tumour a name or not which I can't quite remember now but she called it Tallulah. Or at least she called it Tallulah for a while and then I think, if you give a tumour a name, you give it an identity and that in itself implies both character and separateness from yourself but of course the tumour is part of yourself and so it's not separate from you, so I think she went through a phase of calling it Tallulah.

INTERVIEWER: Okay, so that feels I think two very different sorts of uses of language in a way or I'm not really sure that I'm saying that right, that the Tigger pills was having a bit of laugh.

VA: Yes.

INTERVIEWER: Tallulah actually became more sinister?

VA: Yes, the Tigger pills was a joke, it was a way of dealing with her bounciness when neither of us...

INTERVIEWER: And it was three o'clock in the morning...

VA: Yes and it was a bit wearisome but it was okay because you know it's the Tigger pills that are making you do that. Tallulah was something much darker and much more sinister. I didn't want the tumour to have a name and an identity but it was up to Jane. It was Jane's tumour and if Jane wanted to call it Tallulah then that was up to her but I don't think it was something that went on for that long. It was as I say, a sort of phase.

(*Interview Four, 27 August 2013*)

The reference to Dennis Potter is to the last interview the playwright had with Melvyn Bragg when he knew he was dying from pancreatic cancer. In a wide-ranging discussion, Potter reveals that he had named his tumour Rupert, after the media magnate, Rupert Murdoch, whom he despised (Bragg, 2007). Although there is some anecdotal evidence of people choosing to name their tumours, particularly it seems for brain cancers, I can find no actual research on patient personalisation of their tumours. There is increasing interest in personalised medicine, especially with regard to genomics, although person-specific or individualised care is not in itself something new (Offit, 2011). Within the alternative therapy and self-help health movement there appears to be some belief that naming or at least focusing on your tumour can direct healing forces to it but there is of course no empirical evidence for such a view.

The origin of the name in this context is uncertain but is most likely in reference to the character, Tallulah, in the British musical *Bugsy Malone* and made famous in the 1976 film version by a young Jodie Foster singing 'My name is Tallulah'.[4] So the name was used in conversation between us and then only for a time, Jane never used it in either blog posts or email. Now, I wonder if it seemed to resonate more with me especially when I was researching the visual appearance of ovarian tumours. During the illness, I did not dwell on the tumour and its growth but I was very conscious of the physical effect it was having on Jane's body.

Our experience of health care was completely different. Jane had only been to hospital as an out patient or visitor, enjoying good health until this illness. I was a nurse with many years of hospital practice. Jane had little familiarity with complementary and alternative medicine (CAM)[5] until she met me. I had been dabbling with various aspects for many years before settling on diet, yoga and health supplements. Consequently we believed ourselves to be better for the regime, although a healthy diet and regular exercise are considered more than adequate. But any suggestions that there might be other, complementary therapies that could help Jane is met with refusal for fear of interfering with treatment. However, Jane reappraises her trenchant position after the cathartic meeting with the herbalist when it is suggested there might be something she could *do* to feel calmer when faced with difficult situations. It is on this basis Jane then agrees to see a psychologist to help her with some relaxation techniques:

> It was a mid-evening appointment which was fine and I took her and just waited. I found that quite challenging because apart from the CT scan and when I would leave her for an hour when she was having chemo, she basically wasn't out of my sight and so this was mysterious. Somebody else was doing things with her so I just had to trust and let her do her thing. She came out of the session and on the way home talked a little bit about it, that the woman had been very helpful. It hadn't been a talking therapy, [the psychologist] just talked to her about a visualisation and helped Jane to find something, a visual metaphor that she could use when she started to feel stressed or uncomfortable. What Jane chose was a rock and it was a rock that she could climb onto. So she might be in fast moving water but there was this rock and she could get onto the rock and then feel entirely calm. After she had this session she would talk about sitting on her rock or 'I'm just going to get on my rock' and she could take herself to this place and be much calmer.
>
> The whole experience of first seeing the herbalist and then seeing the counsellor had shifted something huge for Jane. She now had taken ownership of what was happening to her and she was in control and I felt that I was able then to take instruction from her. It wasn't that I was dictating what happened but I found myself asking her all the time 'what do you want to do', 'how do you want to do this' and so on. Previously I think she had just let me say 'we're doing this', 'we're doing that'.
>
> *(Interview Four, 27 August 2013)*

Jane has not necessarily appeared passive in facing her diagnosis, yet it is difficult for her to actively engage in treatment. All she needs to do is ingest or be injected with the various drugs of the regime. We even joked that it was just as well that it was her who was ill as I would have never have sat still long enough for the drugs to be infused. But after the meeting with the psychologist, an aura of calm appears to have replaced what I had perceived as Jane's denial of her situation. Whilst this denial may have been a partial adaptation response (Goldbeck, 1997) it is only now that an actual adjustment has occurred. One possible interpretation could be that of cognitive adaptation theory (CAT) which proposes that threatening events or situations can be addressed through an adjustment process that restores meaning, control and self-esteem (Taylor, 1983). It is through maintaining illusion which "requires looking at the known facts in a particular light, because a different slant would yield a less positive picture" (Taylor, 1983: 1161). A study of women with breast cancer considered the possibly detrimental effect of having an illusion disproved but concluded that CAT "views people as adaptable, self-protective, and functional in the face of setbacks" (Taylor, 1983: 1170).

More recently, similar conclusions have been reached and also questioned the continued reliance, at least in the USA, on a model of adjustment for those dying of cancer that does not fully capture quality of life (Christianson et al., 2013). The authors refer specifically to the model proposed by Kubler-Ross with its five stages of dying: denial, anger, bargaining, depression and acceptance (Kubler-Ross, 1970). Writing in a compassionate style, her focus and emphasis was on the need for realistic acceptance of terminal illness. At the time it would have appealed to those working in the early days of the hospice movement when there was little guidance and few resources. She wanted those caring for the terminally ill to "take a good hard look at our own attitude to death and dying before we can sit quietly and without anxiety next to a terminally ill patient" (Kubler-Ross, 1970: 240). However, the model has been criticised for being too neat and tidy, too American and more a vision of the good death than a model derived from empirical evidence (Barry & Yuill, 2011). The success of her book, *Death and Dying*, led in later years to more personal criticism and claims of arrogant self-aggrandisement (Parkes, 2013). Yet, in the introduction to the 40th edition, the thanato-sociologist Allan Kellehear describes the text as "one of the most important humanitarian works on the care of the dying" (Kellehear, 2009: vii). While there can be little argument that the text did, and continues to, facilitate dialogue about death and dying, such a staged process-oriented interpretation of an individual's situation may be as detrimental as helpful through its notion of a 'right way' to die.

Returning to the narrative and the effect of Jane's visualisation training:

INTERVIEWER: So from being sort of passive and in the back seat, she moved forward into the front seat or the driving sear or something like that?

VA: Yes, it really was a sort of turning point, she was taking over.

INTERVIEWER: And you mention it in relation to that you in a sense had to say what do you want to do but how did she come forward, I mean how did that show itself in other ways? In her demeanour, how she held herself?

VA: I think, it's almost as if she had been carrying this burden on her back and she put it down and sat back and was calmer, was more relaxed. I think we started to talk more in terms of we were going to make the best of what we had and we would do things for as long as she felt able to do them and we would do whatever it was she wanted to do. She should say the places she wanted to visit, the things she wanted to see and that it was as if she had become royalty, that she could command whatever she wanted and her subjects would obey her every wish, but it was up to her to say what it was she wanted.

INTERVIEWER: And so trying to get a feel for how she did that, she moved from the back to the front because I really noticed there is a difference.

VA: She glided, the slightly panicky, frightened almost child-like look had gone from her eyes and it was as if she had glided into this more graceful, calmer state ... There was a more relaxed attitude and approach to it, we were just going take it easy.

INTERVIEWER: So, the veneer of optimism, was that still there then?

VA: It was a different optimism.

INTERVIEWER: Right.

VA: I suppose it was a more real. Finally we understood or there was a shared understanding that this might not be going to get better, this might not be going away, that maybe her time was much more limited than she had first thought. She had initially thought that she would have seven years because they would do the treatment as they'd said and she would still have a few years and that horizon had changed quite dramatically. It was down to one to two years and even at that it was under review, but she was facing that and accepting it in a very different way than from what she had been able to do at the point of diagnosis and the initial treatment.

INTERVIEWER: This isn't part of the storyboard[6] but it feels like a sort of balance has shifted between the two of you?

VA: Yes, it was almost as if she was more like her old self, she was back in control. I had had to take over for about three months and literally hold everything and although I still had to do that in a physical sense, it was down to me to run the household, she was now my queen. She was calling the shots, she was in control and that was a more comfortable relationship despite all the underlying discomfort of her illness.

INTERVIEWER: But I'm getting a real kind of sense of when you said Jane had been carrying a burden and she put it down, that something had clearly shifted and had made room for other things.

VA: Yes, I hadn't particularly thought of it as that but I think that's right. Until that turning point, it was entirely the burden of the tumour and the carrying of it. She was physically conscious of it, she could feel it, she could feel what she described as this brick but then her focus shifted from the brick to the rock.

(Interview Four, 27 August 2013)

This passage suggests that Jane, on learning her diagnosis and subsequent treatment plan, may have been in what has been described as uncertain open awareness:

> when confronted with bad news, the patient or family member disregards the negative aspects and holds on to the chance of a good outcome … People in this context do not dismiss the possibility of a fatal outcome, but they prefer the uncertainty of not understanding exactly what is going on. They pick and choose in each message; hope is more important than a certainty of death.
>
> *(Timmermans, 1994: 330)*

Timmermans had intended to use awareness theory (Glaser & Strauss, 1966) in this introspective ethnographic study of emotional coping mechanisms employed by patients and their relatives when faced with information of terminal illness. However, the author's mother became terminally ill during the study resulting in an additional, powerful dimension to an early example of autoethnography. Timmermans (1994) refined awareness theory, the idea that knowledge of a terminal diagnosis is either closed or unknown to the patient, and possibly their family, or open and known to all. His interpretation expands open awareness to three discernible types:

- Suspended open awareness: ignore the information
- Uncertain open awareness: preference for uncertainty, choose favourable messages, privilege hope
- Active open awareness: full acceptance of the message with appropriate actions

While Timmermans (1994) claims that the emotional shock of diagnosis requires its information to undergo adaptive processing before it can be fully accepted, Mamo (1999) argues that it is not simply cognitive information processing but the emotional effort in comprehending new knowledge that obscures awareness. Since the formal diagnosis, I had understood the implications of the disease but I also knew Jane remained in a state of hopeful optimism that the treatment would be effective. Hope is a ubiquitous concept in any discussion of cancer and life-limiting illness, as perhaps is optimism. Perhaps it is not unreasonable to surmise that people will react differently depending on their dispositional optimism. This can be defined "in terms of the favourability of a person's generalised outcome expectancy" (Bryant & Cvengros, 2004: 232). In other words, an optimistic person will look on the bright side despite a gloomy diagnosis. Hope has been defined as "the sum of perceived capabilities to produce routes to desired goals, along with the perceived motivation to use those routes" (Snyder, 2000: 8).

However, in reviews of the concept of hope in the palliative care context, both Clayton et al. (2008) and Kylmä et al. (2009) ignore Snyder's work and cite a nursing definition of hope as a "confident yet uncertain expectation of achieving future good, which, to the hoping person, is realistically possible and personally significant" (Dufault & Martocchio, 1985: 380). While not unreasonable, this does seem devoid of self efficacy in attaining or maintaining hope. The hopeful person passively waits for something good to happen. In the context of a cancer diagnosis that would be cure or prolonged survival (Clayton et al., 2008). Snyder's (2000) theory of hope is predicated on a trilogy of goals (desired outcome), pathways (routes), and agency (motivation). This seems to be a more useful approach in the context of person-centred care. In a study of the actual use of the word 'hope' by dying patients, Eliott and Olver (2007) suggest that as a noun, hope is limited to the objective reality of the medical world, where there is no hope. As a verb, action is implied, there is something to be done *by* and not *to* the patient. This positive interpretation provides the patient with agency to focus on life and not their imminent death. Yet this approach to hope can accentuate a focus on the future which is hard for someone with a terminal diagnosis and creates a tension. This can be resolved by shifting the focus away from the future to now by living in the present.

The shift from passivity to active engagement suggested by this interpretation of hope provides an explanation for Jane's positive reappraisal of her situation. Publicly, Jane continues with her face-work (Goffman, 1955), using poise to counteract her embarrassment of being ill, but occasionally her guard slips and she expresses her real feelings. In an email to the scientific cousin she reflects on the conventional treatment regime and her own views:

> I am now – following discussion with the herbalist and consultation of quite a lot of research – back on my full programme of supplements. The medical profession in this country will not sanction many of these because they have not done enough double blind trials to be absolutely sure they do not conflict with chemotherapy. In the US they have done quite a lot of work confirming how complementary medicines actually support the chemotherapy. Much of the received wisdom from the medical profession is very tentative, they will not do or recommend anything outside NICE guidelines – the medics keep everything tight and rigid so they are in control. That's the thing that I found most difficult to cope with in the first few months of my treatment – being so scared of doing anything that wasn't officially sanctioned, following every instruction to the letter, in case I did something that made the chemo not work. I have come to realise that it's not because I took mushroom complex or ate yoghurt that the tumour didn't shrink very much – it's because it was a bloody big mass in the first place and chemotherapy is a very blunt instrument.
> (Jane's email to cousin, 4 October 2011)

The blunt crudeness of the chemotherapy is making its presence felt in Jane's blood and her haemoglobin (Hb) had finally become too low for comfort. She had in fact complained of feeling a little short of breath when we were hill-walking one day but I thought it was the effort of trudging up a steep section. Although we are now settled in the flat and there is a rhythm to daily life, it does not always go according to plan:

> Chemo day and we were late as we got snarled in traffic around the tram works. Heard yesterday Hb is down to 97 so they want to transfuse 2 units on Monday. Both a bit freaked by this but mutual resolve it's for the best.
> (Personal diary, 30 September 2011)

Being a blood donor had never been an issue for either of us and we had both been regular donors in the past. But giving blood is one thing, receiving someone else's is another matter entirely. My first reaction was that she should have mine but it is a different group notwithstanding the practical and ethical issues. We both felt conflicted knowing she needed the transfusion but ambivalent about its provenance. The scientific cousin is at hand to discuss the issue:

> JANE: I had to go back in yesterday to have two units of blood. Took about 5 hours. They've been threatening me with needing a transfusion since July and we had managed to keep the haemoglobin just above the red line until last week when it fell to 89. So now I'm feeling particularly perky today – and much better colour :)

COUSIN: Glad the blood transfusion's done you some good, you were looking a little pale in one of your pictures but that might have been because you were tired, or in Scotland. What blood type are you?

JANE: My blood type is O+ so they didn't have much trouble with the cross-match. My Dad is O+ and Mum B+ and the great joke when we were young was that we'd have BO. They kept checking my temp every 15 mins yesterday to make sure I didn't have a reaction to someone else's blood. I had convinced myself it used to belong to a nice Edinburgh lady who never smoked or drank very much (didn't do intravenous drugs, or consort with hepatitis sufferers, or eat dodgy meat products, or have multiple sexual partners…) and on that basis I had no adverse reaction whatsoever.

(Jane's email with cousin, 4 October 2011)

Despite searching the literature, no references have been found regarding the emotional aspects or indeed any others in terms of *receiving* donated blood. There is a wealth of evidence on topics ranging from the altruism of blood donation (Titmuss, 1971) to issues of organ donor identity and recipient indebtedness. Yet the blood transfusion episode is a struggle as another body boundary is crossed. The blunt irony of treatment that has destroyed perfectly healthy blood cells now demands alien blood to course through Jane only to be decimated by the next wave of chemotherapy.

Living

In the last story of this chapter, our lives continue to be dominated by a steady stream of appointments as we dance between the GP surgery, the chemotherapy ward and the x-ray department while also making excited preparations for Christmas. My brother and sister with their partners are joining us for a family celebration of closed awareness. We all know and tacitly understand it will be Jane's last. But before the celebrations can begin, Jane has more appointments, the first being at the surgery for a flu vaccination:

VA: One of the practice nurses said that because I was Jane's primary carer, I had to have it as well. I vacillated and said that I wasn't really very sure. She just grabbed me and stuck it in my arm. So I was a mixture of beaten down and furious that she'd made me have it but I wasn't going to do anything that would compromise Jane.

INTERVIEWER: Did that have any impact on Jane?

VA: Well she just laughed, somebody had got one over me.

(Interview Five, 3 September 2013)

Newbury (2009) suggests carer performance may broadly fall into two types: combative and pragmatic. For example, in a combative sense, a carer may feel angry and the need for control, while a more pragmatic style would be to cope and deal with events. The archetypal response to a cancer diagnosis is that of a battle, something to be beaten, to conquer, to win against the odds. Previously, the great disease fear was tuberculosis (TB), borne with a resigned and romanticised dignity among the rich while being despised as inevitable amongst the squalid poor (Bourdelais, 2006). The account in *The Magic Mountain* (Mann, 2005) of isolated but luxurious care in a Swiss sanatorium[7] is not atypical. Recognised as a contagion for centuries, it was not until the 1940s that a viable treatment for TB was found and subsequently largely contained with effective public health measures (Daniel, 2006).

While battling disease is not specific to cancer as HIV and AIDS have been fought and conquered, it was the Lasker Foundation which first found that declaring 'War on cancer' was a very lucrative strategy (DeVita, 2002). As a result, the implementation of the 1971 US Cancer Act was heavily funded by the Foundation. In its current publicity campaign and fund-raising strategy, Cancer Research UK uses the strap line "We will beat cancer sooner. Join the fight"[8] to marshal an army of volunteers and fund-raisers. These groups undertake many extraordinary sponsored challenges to raise money, often in memory of a loved one lost to cancer. Regrettably there is no space here to explore the economics of health research and the disparity in funding between, for example, cancer and dementia (Siddique, 2013). The language used in the USA to raise funds for their 1971 Cancer Act has resulted in the continuing use of such combative terms in response to cancer, its research and treatment.

Returning to carer performance, Newbury (2009) does not reference an earlier study which explored the husband's experience of caring for a wife receiving chemotherapy (Wilson & Morse, 1991). Using interviews and grounded theory, a three stage model was developed from suspecting something might be wrong (Identifying the threat) to actively participating in their wife's care (Engaging in the fight) to getting through chemotherapy (Becoming a veteran). The terms and writing style may now seem dated and gendered, but the process of adjustment described is helpful in understanding the changing nature of an intimate relationship muddied by disease. This model seems to support Newbury's combative carer style which in turn supports the heroic female death as one of concern and emotional expression (Seale, 1995). However, it is the cancer sufferer who really needs a combative style:

> The Canadian Cancer Society widely publicises the slogan, 'Cancer can be Beaten.' This implies that cancer is a disease that can be fought. This analogy of battling or fighting is an activity one must participate in if one is to win. Thus, fighting is a prerequisite to winning. A further implication in the slogan is: if one fights, then one can be hopeful of beating or curing the cancer. Thus, the fighting process provides hope. Finally, the slogan also places the onus on the 'person' to do battle and win rather than on the caregivers or the therapy.
>
> *(Wilson & Morse, 1991: 83)*

Despite being written more than twenty years ago, such bellicose language continues to influence the response to a cancer diagnosis by both the affected person and their primary carer. Initially, Jane knows there is a fight in progress but it is being done by the health care team, so her response is one of passive acceptance. In turn, her powerlessness is reinforced by the disruptive nature of the treatment and her inability to take ownership of the situation. It is only after the cathartic consultation with the herbalist that she takes command:

> The really big thing is realising that while it's not my fault I have cancer, it is my responsibility to deal with it. My body has done this to itself – and only my body can undo it, or contain and control it. With whatever help I choose to give it – medical, chemical, herbal, dietary, and psychological. There are many ways up the mountain. Other people can help – describe the landscape, suggest routes, provide kit and provisions, accompany me for part of the way – but I take the path myself. Knowing this is tremendously empowering. I am not a passive victim, I am in control of my own recovery.
>
> *(Blog post, 'A Different Mindset', 20 September 2011)*

My role is unchanged and I continue to 'buffer' anything I perceive as a threat to Jane's well-being which can now be understood as a common carer response:

> 'Buffering' was a process by which husbands filtered and reduced the stresses of day-to-day living to protect their wives. ... The buffering process involved two active components: constant vigilance and cognitive action. Constant vigilance consisted of watching his wife's response to chemotherapy and her interactions with others. Cognitive action involved the interpretation of his perceptions, judging whether his wife was in a harmful situation and then planning an action designed to buffer.
>
> *(Wilson & Morse, 1991: 80)*

By now we have a regular routine when Jane goes for treatment. I was aware at the time that my behaviour went beyond just 'buffering' as I generally got between Jane and whatever might be going to be done to her. I thought of this as 'guarding' when, for example, I would walk slightly ahead of Jane, with my arm out in front of her. That way, I could fend off any unwanted collisions or people being too near to her space. But it is more difficult to buffer conversations.

> In a really busy ward like a chemotherapy unit there isn't a lot of time but A [favourite nurse] would make time to come and sit. What was particularly special about A was that on one occasion she was sitting talking to us both and she said to Jane, 'you know we can't make you better' and we both said yes we knew. Actually she said 'you know we can't cure you' and we said yes, we understood that this was only going to shrink things, it wasn't going to kill everything or make the tumour completely go away. Nobody else really had

those kind of discussions but I suspect A had sensed something in Jane about the extent to which she was coping with it.

(*Interview Five, 3 September 2013*)

On this occasion I remember feeling awkward at the exchange but accepted it might be helpful for this particular nurse to be honest and frank with Jane. The breezy positivism employed by the majority of the health care team was a cause of frustration as we were both aware of darker realities. Nevertheless, the truthful sincerity was hard to hear.

INTERVIEWER: What was the response to that statement of 'you know we can't cure you'?

VA: I think at the time we both just said yes we understood, we knew that but I found it quite hard. I knew that they couldn't cure Jane but nobody had actually said that. I did feel that they weren't being entirely honest with us and that part of Jane's difficulty in coming to terms with the seriousness of her situation was that she was being carried along by this wave of enthusiasm from the oncologists for treatment.

INTERVIEWER: How did she respond to that statement from A. Can you remember?

VA: I don't think she said anything, I think there was just a look in her eyes that said that she knew, she didn't want to talk about it now. We didn't talk about it a great deal, as I remember.

INTERVIEWER: With the nurses or with each other?

VA: With each other.

INTERVIEWER: What didn't you talk about a great deal, the getting better bit?

VA: The not getting better bit. I think I tried very much to keep up this positive thing of making the most of what we had and the best of each day. We were just going through this process, this production line of chemo in the hope they would be able to do something in the Spring. We were still hopeful of that and even though they couldn't cure her, they could make things a lot better or at least that was what we believed.

INTERVIEWER: Okay, I just have this sense of that being a very kind of potent moment.

VA: Yes, I think that's right but I think it was probably more potent for me. I think I would have heard it in a very different way from how Jane heard it. I heard it as the reality, that it was crossing that line between what the nurses and the doctors talk about and what they tell the family. I felt that A, knowing that I had been a nurse, was respecting that and was trusting me to know the truth, but Jane would almost certainly have heard it slightly differently or perhaps not quite so as emphatically as I did.

(*Interview Five, 3 September 2013*)

It is possible that I needed someone in the team to say that they could not cure Jane and for her to hear what I knew. Perhaps I had been guarding myself from the truth and what the chemo nurse really recognised was my need for it to be revealed. Our preparations for attending a chemo session are meticulous and include not just the provision of respective lunches and snacks, but also Jane's apparel: lucky stripy socks and a humorous tee-shirt. Perhaps this particular nurse has noticed our 'performance' and the positive nature of our demeanour. Concerned that we do not appreciate or understand the seriousness of the situation, she decides to address the issue. This accords with Copp's finding that putting on a brave and cheery face could be "perceived as behaviour not expected of a person in her situation" (Copp, 1996: 195). Consequently, a more astute and compassionate nurse might use such an observation as a cue to explore the emotional and cognitive aspects of a patient's situation. By now we are in a relatively comfortable place as Jane describes:

> That's three months we've been here now, and we are feeling very settled. [Veronica] remarked the other day that we have found contentment, which may seem odd given the health circumstances, but is a pretty accurate assessment of how we feel, and the life we are living. Tests and hospital visits are accommodated into work and play without governing or obsessing us.
> *(Blog Post, 'Fair to Middling', 7 October 2011)*

We have learnt the dance of the chemotherapy routine and mastered the shift in tempo to weekly sessions interspersed with blood tests and scans. Or so we thought. Jane's blood is now showing definite signs of wear and tear, despite the previous blood transfusion. The regular destruction of blood cells and the time interval between poisonings is insufficient for the cells to be replenished. Chemotherapy-induced myelosuppression is known to be the most common toxicity resulting from chemotherapy (Kurtin, 2012). Its effects can be obviated to some extent by the use of combination therapies as with the treatment protocol of Paclitaxel and Carboplatin for Jane. However, Paclitaxel is also known to carry a high risk of myleotoxicity. The general response to signs of such toxicity is to either delay or reduce the dose of the cytotoxic agents but this may also limit the therapeutic potential of the treatment (Kurtin, 2012). We are aware of the risks associated with chemotherapy but unprepared when myelosuppression inevitably occurs.

INTERVIEWER: We're getting ready to go for the chemo again and then A [favourite nurse] phones to say platelets were low and you start off that by saying it was a bit of a weird day. What does weird mean?
VA: We'd got into a rhythm of one day a week for three weeks going for chemo. It started the day before with going for the blood tests at the GP surgery. The hospital saw that her platelets were low and [favourite nurse] said 'you need to come in early, we need to check your bloods and then it depends whether you'll get chemo or not'. So we went in to wait for an hour for the blood result to come back. I didn't want Jane to wait in [the ward] where everybody else was getting chemo, I wanted her to go over to the Maggie's Centre so she

wasn't caught up in it. But she wanted to wait there. The result came back and the platelets were even lower than they had been the day before so there was no way she was having chemo. So you would think that was one week that I don't have to feel awful for two or three days but of course Jane interpreted that as she'd failed a test.

(Interview Five, 3 September 2013)

In fact her reaction is similar to that previously when her bodily response to chemo was poor and the regime was increased "Like not doing as well as I think I should have at my chemo exam and somehow letting myself, and others, down" (Blog post, 'A Different Mindset', day 98). Until this point we have successfully assimilated Jane's illness and treatment into the flow of our daily lives thereby offsetting any biographical disruption (Bury, 1982) and restoring a degree of harmony (Rasmussen & Elverdam, 2007). This is different from the previous occasion when her haemoglobin was low and the transfusion was arranged as a separate treatment. Although we know why a close check is being kept on the status of Jane's blood, we are unprepared for the effect of 'failing' a blood test prior to chemotherapy. For Jane it is traumatic as I note the following day "J a bit washed out after the angst of yesterday" (Personal diary, day 130). The physical effect of no cytotoxic treatment seems to be almost worse than actually having it. Bury's theory of biographical disruption has been further developed to accommodate a fracture to the narrative. A sense of well-being is felt when narrative form is equal to biographical flow or the continuity of daily life. However "maintaining continuity was draining: exhaustion precipitated fracture and thus need for external help to restore continuity" (Reeve et al., 2010: 178). For Jane the continuity of the chemotherapy narrative is disrupted by the failed blood test and she feels 'exhausted' and needs my support to recover.

The following week there is another CT scan and on this occasion "all went well – not quite such an ordeal this time" (Personal diary, day 139). Jane knows what to do and is better able to pace drinking the litre of contrast medium. There has also been some reduction in her abdominal swelling so the additional volume does not cause so much discomfort. We then discover an aspect of the intensive chemotherapy regime we did not appreciate: failing a blood test means a week is missed and not just postponed. We arrive for the unscheduled session the following week only to find we have both misunderstood the process.

I knew that we hadn't done something wrong but it was such a disappointment for Jane. She did have to psych herself up for the chemo, I knew that. It was a performance, it was an ordeal because there were such swings of being high from the steroids and then just the tiring nature of sitting still for six hours and having all this stuff in you. Then the feeling of everything having stopped the next day and then the feeling you've got bad flu.

(Interview Five, 3 September 2013)

In this situation it was neither biographical disruption nor temporal discord that was the issue but a failure to understand the "ruling relations" (Smith, 2005: 10) of the treatment regime and hospital procedures. We were overwhelmed with treatment leaflets, guidelines and cancer charity pamphlets. Despite our mutual capacity to understand much of this information, we had both failed to grasp the nuances of this particular dance. In response I attempt some buffering behaviour (Wilson & Morse, 1991): "had fish fingers for tea to cheer her up" (Personal diary, day 143). After the scan there is a follow-up visit to the oncology clinic but on this occasion there was a different consultant, a cheery woman; smiles all round.

INTERVIEWER: Did her gender make any difference?

VA: I'm not sure, she talked about had we looked at the Ovacome site because she had been the medical advisor for that and I think we both said no because neither of us found these cancer support sites particularly helpful. But she was very enthusiastic and I think Jane said she would then have a look at it. Whether her gender made any difference, I think I wanted it to but it didn't.

INTERVIEWER: I wondered, was there any sense from Jane that things might be improving, any change in symptoms or anything like that; was it possible for her to notice?

VA: I think she was wary because she had been feeling better the last time only to be told that the chemo wasn't having that much effect and so she was a bit more guarded.

(Interview Five, 3 September 2013)

The scan report is unequivocal:

> When compared with the previous recent scan, there has been a definite reduction in the volume of the ascites. However the nodal metastatic disease and the pelvic tumour bulk mass appear similar in size and extent, although this is difficult to quantify, particularly in the pelvis. No new disease sites seen.
> *(Hospital CT scan report, 1 November 2011)*

The improvement is that there is less fluid in Jane's abdomen, which she has noticed, but in reality the chemotherapy had not affected the tumour; growth had been halted but not reduced. Nevertheless, the oncologist is keen to continue with the chemotherapy and for a review by the surgeon. Jane now takes a more active interest in her health:

> I started to feel quite strongly – and conversations with many other people backed this up – that my body was telling me it would cope much better with the side-effects of the treatment if I gave it a bit more support. In the US, the use of complementary medicine alongside chemotherapy (not as an alternative) is increasingly supported. There's growing evidence that many vitamins and

supplements not only help to counteract the side-effects, but can potentiate the primary effect i.e. killing the cancer.

So I've been taking lots of carefully researched and selected vitamins and minerals. That's when I started on weekly chemo. It's also when tests indicate the tumour really started to shrink. So far so good. Fresh air and exercise continue to be vital strategies. I'm a walking biology lesson, fascinated by my weekly haematology and blood chemistry print-outs. I often wish I could discuss this with my Dad, I think he would have enjoyed that!

(Blog post 'Coping with Chemo', 20 November 2011)

Jane's comment "when tests indicate the tumour really started to shrink" refers to the tumour marker CA-125 which had been measured regularly since diagnosis. In the previous chapter, its continued rise after treatment started was noted, but now it was falling. This finding is not in itself unusual as the marker is a difficult and controversial indicator, with up to 50% false negative results (Marcus et al., 2014). The test involves the detection of a protein in the blood which is secreted by ovarian cancer cells; in simple terms, if the tumour is active, the protein will be exuded. While Jane interprets the marker's fall as the tumour shrinking, the CT scan shows otherwise. The tumour is not shrinking, it is merely dormant.

Over the next few weeks the dance between the GP surgery, the chemo ward and the rest of our lives continues uneventfully. Jane's blood profile is closely monitored and although borderline, she receives a complete three week treatment cycle. Preparations for our Christmas visitors progress and I create a bedouin tent-come-spare room in the attic. Another review meeting is scheduled, this time with the surgeon as promised by the woman oncologist at the previous clinic meeting.

INTERVIEWER: So you went for an audience with the surgeon, now that's a very particular word so how important was this meeting?

VA: Well it was quite important. This was the first time Jane had seen the surgeon since the initial diagnosis.

INTERVIEWER: So you say that this was all a bit strange and uncertain [referring to storyboard], so what was happening for you in this meeting?

VA: We were starting to be aware that there was a big question mark over whether surgery would be possible. The surgeon had always been very clear he wasn't going to go in and just start rummaging about doing stuff if he wasn't confident that he wasn't going to make Jane worse. So it was partly as a kind of reassurance that we must continue with the chemotherapy.

INTERVIEWER: When you say reassurance, was he reassuring you or were you being reassured, I mean?

VA: Well I think that was what was supposed to happen but we weren't really reassured because I think we were trying to get straight answers and in the end he [the surgeon] just printed off the scan report and gave it to us. We didn't believe the oncologists because we would get a copy of the blood results from the GP and we knew what the tumour marker, the CA 125 was. We knew

how much it was coming down or not and it wasn't falling anything like as fast enough, as it should've done and they would say to us 'oh it's only a number, it doesn't matter'.
INTERVIEWER: Okay, and he gave you the scan report?
VA: Yes, he printed it off.
INTERVIEWER: So did he discuss it with you or did he just give it to you?
VA: Well he said it's difficult to know. Basically the scan report says not much has improved, there's a bit less fluid but there doesn't appear to be much shrinkage.

(Interview Five, 3 September 2013)

At the time of the interviews I did not have access to Jane's health records and believed that the referral to the surgeon was made by Jane's usual oncologist. It was only when I saw the records that I realised it was the woman oncologist who had made the referral. It is difficult to know how or why this made any difference, but I sensed a certain frustration for the surgeon. Clearly the tumour had not shrunk and it was most unlikely he could do anything surgical, but by giving us the scan report, he could at least be completely honest. We had been trying to get straight answers to straight questions both when Jane attended for chemotherapy and in discussion with the clinical nurse specialist (CNS). Whoever was asked in the oncology team always made light of Jane's situation and refused to be drawn on the tumour marker results.

It was not that we did not trust or respect the oncology team, we knew they were doing their best in very difficult circumstances, but we needed the candour of the surgeon. He recognised this and trusted us to cope with the stark reality of the CT scan report. We knew from his energetic reaction to Jane's condition when they first met that he would do anything he could to make her better, but only if it did not make her worse. Long gone were the days of going in and taking out as much of the bad bits as you could and then re-plumbing whatever was left and other ghastly memories. His feelings are clear in his letter to Jane's GP:

This patient was reviewed today. She has had minimal response in her CT interval scans and a fairly partial response to her CA-125. However, she is young, slim, very fit and we will organise a diagnostic laparoscopy at the beginning of January to determine whether she is surgically operable, however, I have feeling that this will probably involve the colorectal surgeons and possibly involve the urological surgeons.

I will take this opportunity to write to [colorectal surgeon] and ask her if she has any free dates for a joint procedure which will involve probably most of a morning or an afternoon list and possibly the formation of a colostomy or an ileostomy of which the patient is fully aware.

Ps: Dear [colorectal surgeon],

This patient is absolutely delightful, she is young, she is certainly fairly majorly compromised with her current underlying ovarian cancer and I would appreciate if you could perhaps consider a joint procedure in early February for a fairly extensive mid line laparotomy and debulking procedure.

(Letter from surgeon to GP, 6 December 2011)

My recollections are a further illustration of the ongoing issue of awareness. The surgeon confirms that Jane is fully aware of her condition and of what to expect from surgery. His interpretation of the response to chemotherapy is 'minimal' from the CT scans and 'partial' in the CA-125 results. His findings can be contrasted with the woman oncologist's letter to him, where she notes:

> I met with this lady following the MDM on behalf of [usual oncologist] and clinically she is feeling much better indeed. She feels her abdomen has become a lot less distended and that she is eating well and there is less pelvic pain. We plan to continue with a further two months of the weekly chemotherapy, but would be grateful if you could see her in the interim to discuss possible surgery thereafter. We appreciate that this may not be possible. She may need laparoscopic assessment again, but also appreciate that surgery, if it does go ahead, will require some co-origination.
>
> *(Oncologist letter to surgeon copied to GP, 10 November 2011)*

These different styles in interpretation and in the encounters we had with the clinicians confirm Furber's findings in her doctoral study of the exchange of information in the advanced cancer setting. Doctors use a variety of styles to give and discuss "sharing uncomfortable news" ranging from "fudging the truth" to "mutual understanding" (Furber, 2010: 199). For us, the oncologists tended to fudge, while the surgeon engaged in mutual understanding. I do not want to appear overly critical of the oncology team but we did have a sense of being played between the two clinical specialties, especially when the surgeon had expressed a slight frustration at being asked to review Jane's progress. We had the sense that he had made his views clear in the most recent MDM, having referred to the 'dreadful burden' in the first MDM. Initially the lead oncologist gave a frank account of the discussion at our first meeting, which he reported in his letter to the GP "The lady and her partner were already well up to speed with the situation and the precarious situation that she is in" (Oncologist letter to GP, 21 July 2011).

Now this awareness seemed to have waned and the focus has shifted from the disease itself to Jane's clinical appearance, emphasising the positive 'she is feeling much better indeed'. But this upbeat response was written by the woman oncologist, who does not know Jane so well as the lead oncologist she usually sees. There is a frustratingly gendered issue here: the men (the surgeon and the usual oncologist) were "telling it straight" while the women (the other oncologist and the CNS) were telling it slant (Long, 1999: 37). Judy Long took the idea of women putting a slant on telling something from an Emily Dickinson poem:

> Tell all the truth but tell it slant
> Success in circuit lies
> Too bright for our infirm Delight
> The truth's superb surprise
> As lightening to the Children eased
> With explanation kind
> The truth must dazzle gradually
> Or every man be blind
> (Dickinson, 1976: 506, 1129)

This was the 'explanation kind' for the 'truth must dazzle gradually'. Yet what we wanted was directness and not just information which we then had to frame and reach conclusions for ourselves (Borrelli, 2002). It would be unfair to criticise the oncologists for trying to retain optimism in the face of what might otherwise be perceived as a hopeless case. Nevertheless it is notoriously difficult for clinicians to get the balance right over time and in each patient encounter (Innes & Payne, 2009; Furber et al., 2014). Our situation though, was subtly different from the encounters discussed and reviewed in these studies. We were fully aware of Jane's situation but were having difficulty reconciling the enthusiasm of some members of the oncology team with the empirical evidence of the poor response to treatment. Another interpretation could be that the women health professionals felt they recognised in Jane a need for a slant which was more important than my demands for straight talking. If I was blind to her needs, they were not, she needed time to assimilate the truth.

We do not dwell on this sorry state for long as Christmas and the arrival of our visitors is fast approaching. Time for some mutual face-work (Goffman, 1955) and a group hug from the circle of love of our nearest and dearest. Jane continues to have chemo, but also needed another blood transfusion. The actual day everyone is scheduled to arrive is also a chemo day. However (as luck would have it?), the hospital phone to say Jane's platelets are borderline and she needs to go in earlier to have them rechecked. I note the complicated dance for the day:

> Logistics day – flights on time so dropped J for bloods then to airport. [Sister & her husband] fine, back to [hospital] to collect J. Not long back when [brother & girlfriend] arrived! [Hospital] phoned – platelets no change so no chemo. Then GP phoned – muddle with the marker – it's going back up – not so good :(
>
> (Personal diary, 23 December 2011)

When asked about this episode, I recall:

> Our own GP had phoned to ask how Jane was and to say she was sorry that the tumour marker had started to go back up. I just remember standing in the kitchen and saying to my sister, that was it, it was going in the wrong

direction and we'd given it our best shot but it wasn't working as we'd hoped but that it was really important that we made the best of everything for Jane. And Jane understood, just as I did, that this wasn't good news but I think she just wanted to park it. She still had the prospect of the diagnostic lap being done in the Spring and everybody had just arrived and she just wanted to enjoy everybody's company and forget about it. Enough, there was nothing we could do then and what we could do was have a good Christmas.

(Interview Six, 10 September 2013)

This polarisation of the joy of the family arriving and the dismal news from the GP was difficult for us both to bear at the time. We never understood why the GP decided to call and there is no mention of it in Jane's primary health care record. It was just one of those unfortunate incidents which was meant with the best of intentions but was also ill-timed. Equally, the timing, while not perfect, was almost fortuitous as it did galvanise everyone to make every effort for a harmonious celebration.

It was, we generally decreed, the best Christmas ever. [We] had resolved when we came back to Scotland in March that we would have a wee cosy place where [my siblings and their partners] could come and we could all be together for Christmas. The plan worked. The circle of love came home. It was great.

(Blog post 'Festive Family Favourites', 12 January 2012)

This chapter has recounted and analysed the treatment phase of the Illness Period. The initial enthusiasm of the quick response by the health care team has ended with the disappointment of the chemotherapy failure being offset by the joy of a family Christmas at home. The next chapter, the last in *The Dance to Death*, relates the gradual decline in Jane's physical well-being and culminates with her death.

Notes

1 The symbolic significance of yew trees will soon become clear.
2 See WHO Global Burden of Disease web site: www.who.int/topics/global_burden_of_disease/en/
3 Breast Cancer 1 and Breast Cancer 2 – see Narod & Salmena (2011) for historical overview.
4 See: Mansour, 2005: 60; *Bugsy Malone* (1976) Directed by Alan Parker [Film] UK: Rank Organisation.
5 The US National Center for Complementary and Alternative Medicine (NCCAM) differentiates between therapies which support conventional treatment (complementary) and those which are as '*alternatives*'. In the UK patients are less likely to engage with CAM therapies although those with breast and ovarian cancers are the most likely (Molassiotis et al., 2005; Helpman et al., 2011).
6 This may appear as the interviewer acting as researcher but she was just following her brief to elicit the shared experience and prompting accordingly.

7 I must confess a certain fondness for such a life as my parents, both of whom contracted TB in their early twenties, met while recuperating in a sanatorium.
8 Publicity from 2015 website, see www.cancerresearchuk.org

References

Barry, A-M & Yuill, C (2011) 'Death and dying', in A-M Barry & C Yuill, Eds, *Understanding the Sociology of Health*, London: SAGE Publications Ltd, 305–325

Bates, Erica (1982) 'Doctors and their spouses speak: stress in medical practice', *Sociology of Health & Illness*, 4, 1

Borrelli, Mary Anne (2002) 'Telling it slant: gender roles, power, and narrative style in the first ladies' autobiographies', *Sex Roles*, 47, 7/8, 355–370

Bourdelais, P (2006) *Epidemics Laid Low: A History of What Happened in Rich Countries*, Baltimore, MD: Johns Hopkins University Press

Bragg, Melvyn (2007) 'We tend to forget that life can only be defined in the present tense', *The Guardian*, 12 September

Bryant, Fred B & Cvengros, Jamie A (2004) 'Distinguishing hope and optimism: two sides of a coin, or two separate coins?', *Journal of Social & Clinical Psychology*, 23, 273–302

Bury, Michael (1982) 'Chronic illness as biographical disruption', *Sociology of Health & Illness*, 4, 167–183

Caruth, Cathy (1995) *Trauma: Explorations in Memory*, Baltimore: Johns Hopkins University Press

Catt, S, Fallowfield, L, Jenkins, V, Langridge, C & Cox, A (2005) 'The informational roles and psychological health of members of 10 oncology multidisciplinary teams in the UK', *British Journal of Cancer*, 93, 1092–1097

Christianson, H F, Weis, J M & Fouad, N A (2013) 'Cognitive adaptation theory and quality of life in late-stage cancer patients', *Journal of Psychosocial Oncology*, 31, 266–281

Clayton, J M, Hancock, H, Parker, S, Butow, P N, Walder, S, Carrick, S, Currow, D, Ghersi, D, Glare, P, Hagerty, R, Olver, I N & Tattersall, M H (2008) 'Sustaining hope when communicating with terminally ill patients and their families: a systematic review', *Psycho-Oncology*, 17, 641–659

Copp, Gina (1996) *Facing Impending Death: The Experiences of Patients and their Nurses in a Hospice Setting*, PhD, Oxford: Oxford Brookes University

Daniel, Thomas M (2006) 'The history of tuberculosis', *Respiratory Medicine*, 100, 1862–1870

DeVita, Jr, Vincent T (2002) 'A perspective on the war on cancer', *The Cancer Journal*, 8, 352–356

Dickinson, Emily (1976) *Complete Poems*, London: Faber & Faber

Dufault, K & Martocchio, B C (1985) 'Hope: its spheres and dimensions', *Nursing Clinics of North America*, 20, 379–391

Eliott, Jaklin A & Olver, Ian N (2007) 'Hope and hoping in the talk of dying cancer patients', *Social Science & Medicine*, 64, 1, 138–149

Fallowfield, Lesley (2009) *What is Quality of Life?*, Newmarket: Hayward Medical Communications

Furber, Lynn (2010) *Investigating Interactions: How do Doctors and Patients Experience the Disclosure of Significant Information in the Advanced Cancer Setting and How do these Experiences Enhance Practice?*, PhD thesis, Nottingham: University of Nottingham

Furber, Lynn, Bonas, S, Murtagh, G & Thomas, A (2014) 'Patients' experiences of an initial consultation in oncology: knowing and not knowing', *British Journal of Health Psychology*, 20, 2, 261–273

Gadamer, Hans-Georg (2004) *Truth and Method*, New York: Continuum International Publishing Group Ltd, 2nd edition

Glaser Barney, G & Strauss, Anselm L (1966) *Awareness of Dying*, Chicago: Aldine
Goethe, Johann Wolfgang (2007) *Faust: A Tragedy in Two Parts*, Ware: Wordsworth Classics of World Literature
Goffman, Erving (1955) 'On face-work: an analysis of ritual elements in social interaction', *Psychiatry: Journal for the Study of Interpersonal Processes*, 18, 213–231
Goldbeck, Rainer (1997) 'Denial in physical illness', *Journal of Psychosomatic Research*, 43, 575–593
Helpman, L, Ferguson, S E, Mackean, M, Rana, A, Le, L, Atkinson, M A & Mackay, H (2011) 'Complementary and alternative medicine use among women receiving chemotherapy for ovarian cancer in two patient populations', *International Journal of Gynecological Cancer*, 21, 3, 587–593
Hilton, B Ann, Crawford, John A & Tarko, Michel A (2000) 'Men's perspectives on individual and family coping with their wives' breast cancer and chemotherapy', *Western Journal of Nursing Research*, 22, 4, 438–459
Innes, S & Payne, S (2009) 'Advanced cancer patients' prognostic information preferences: a review', *Palliative Medicine*, 23, 29–39
Jantz, Harold (1953) 'The place of the "eternal-womanly" in Goethe's Faust drama', *PMLA*, 68, 791–805
Jayde, V, Boughton, M & Blomfield, P (2013) 'The experience of chemotherapy-induced alopecia for Australian women with ovarian cancer', *European Journal of Cancer Care*, 22, 503–512
Jung, C G (1971) *Psychological Types*, London: Routledge
Kellehear, Allan (2009) 'Introduction to the 40th anniversary edition', in E Kübler-Ross, Ed., *On Death and Dying: What the Dying Have to Teach Doctors, Nurses, Clergy and their Own Families*, Oxford: Routledge, vii–xviii
Kinderman, W & Syer, K R (2005) *A Companion to Wagner's Parsifal*, London: Camden House
Koszalinski, Rebecca S & Williams, Christine (2012) 'Embodying identity in chemotherapy-induced alopecia', *Perspectives in Psychiatric Care*, 48, 116–121
Kubler-Ross, Elizabeth (1970) *On Death and Dying*, London: Tavistock Publications
Kurtin, Sandra (2012) 'Myeloid toxicity of cancer treatment', *Journal of the Advanced Practitioner in Oncology*, 3, 4
Kylmä, Jari, Duggleby, W, Cooper, D & Molander, G (2009) 'Hope in palliative care: an integrative review', *Palliative & Supportive Care*, 7, 365–377
Long, Judy (1999) *Telling Women's Lives: Subject, Narrator, Reader, Text*, New York: New York University Press
Mamo, Laura (1999) 'Death and dying: confluences of emotion and awareness', *Sociology of Health & Illness*, 21, 13–36
Mansour, David (2005) *From Abba to Zoom: A Pop Culture Encyclopaedia of the Late 20th Century*, Kansas City: Andrews McMeel Publishing
Mann, Thomas (2005) *The Magic Mountain*, London: Everyman's Library
Marcus, Charlotte S, Maxwell, G L, Darcy, K M, Hamilton, C A, & McGuire, W P (2014) 'Current approaches and challenges in managing and monitoring treatment response in ovarian cancer', *Journal of Cancer*, 5, 1, 25–30
Mattingly, Cheryl (1998) 'In search of the good: narrative reasoning in clinical practice', *Medical Anthropology Quarterly*, 12, 273–297
May, C R, Eton, D T, Boehmer, K, Gallacher, K, Hunt, K, MacDonald, S, Mair, F S, May, C M, Montori, V M, Richardson, A, Rogers, A E & Shippee, N (2014) 'Rethinking the patient: using Burden of Treatment Theory to understand the changing dynamics of illness', *BMC Health Services Research*, 14

Mellon, Suzanne & Northouse, Laurel L (2001) 'Family survivorship and quality of life following a cancer diagnosis', *Research in Nursing & Health*, 24, 6, 446–459

Molassiotis, A, Fernadez-Ortega, P, Pud, D, Ozden, G, Scott, J A, Panteli, V, Margulies, A, Browall, M, Magri, M, Selvekerova, S, Madsen, E, Milovics, L, Bruyns, I, Gudmundsdottir, G, Hummerston, S, Ahmad, A M-A, Platin, N, Kearney, N & Patiraki, E (2005) 'Use of complementary and alternative medicine in cancer patients: a European survey', *Annals of Oncology*, 16, 655–663

Montazeri, Ali (2009) 'Quality of life data as prognostic indicators of survival in cancer patients: an overview of the literature from 1982 to 2008', *Health & Quality of Life Outcomes*, 7, 102

Murray, C J L & Lopez, A D (1996) *The Global Burden of Disease: A Comprehensive Assessment of Mortality and Disability from Diseases, Injuries, and Risk Factors in 1990 and Projected to 2020*, Cambridge: Harvard School Of Public Health

Narod, Steven A & Salmena, Leonardo (2011) 'BRCA1 and BRCA2 mutations and breast cancer', *Discovery Medicine*, 12, 445–453

Newbury, Margaret J (2009) *The Carer's Initiation: A Qualitative Study of the Experience of Family Care of the Dying*, Professional Doctorate in Health thesis, Bath: University of Bath

Offit, Kenneth (2011) 'Personalized medicine: new genomics, old lessons', *Human Genetics*, 130, 3–14

Parkes, Colin Murray (2013) 'Elisabeth Kübler-Ross, *On Death and Dying*: a reappraisal', *Mortality*, 18, 94–97

Paus, R, Haslam, I S, Sharov, A A & Botchkarev, V A (2013) 'Pathobiology of chemotherapy-induced hair loss', *The Lancet Oncology*, 14, 2, e50–e59

Ramirez, A J, Graham, J, Richards, M A, Cull, A & Gregory, W M (1996) 'Mental health of hospital consultants: the effects of stress and satisfaction at work', *The Lancet*, 347, 724–728

Rasmussen, Dorte M & Elverdam, Beth (2007) 'Cancer survivors' experience of time: time disruption and time appropriation', *Journal of Advanced Nursing*, 57, 614–622

Reeve, Joanne, Lloyd-Williams, M, Payne, S & Dowrick, C (2010) 'Revisiting biographical disruption: exploring individual embodied illness experience in people with terminal cancer', *Health*, 14, 178–195

Robinson, James C (1986) 'Philosophical origins of the economic valuation of life', *The Milbank Quarterly*, 133–155

Roe, Helen (2011) 'Chemotherapy-induced alopecia: advice and support for hair loss', *British Journal of Nursing*, 20, S4–11

Rosman, Sophia (2004) 'Cancer and stigma: experience of patients with chemotherapy-induced alopecia', *Patient Education & Counseling*, 52, 333–339

Seale, Clive (1995) 'Heroic death', *Sociology*, 29, 4, 597–613

Shand, L K, Brooker, J E, Burney, S, Fletcher, J & Ricciardelli, L A (2014) 'Symptoms of post-traumatic stress in Australian women with ovarian cancer', *Psycho-Oncology*, 24, 2, 190–196

Siddique, H (2013) 'Dementia research funding should be on same footing as cancer, says charity', *The Guardian*, Society, 11 December

SIGN (2013) *Epithelial Ovarian Cancer*, Edinburgh: Scottish Intercollegiate Guidelines Network, 135

Smith, D E (2005) *Institutional Ethnography: A Sociology for People*, Lanham: AltaMira Press

Snyder, C R (2000) 'Hypothesis: There is hope', in C R Snyder, Ed., *Handbook of Hope: Theory, Measures & Applications*, Waltham: Academic Press, 3–21

Stacey, Jackie (1997) *Teratologies: A Cultural Study of Cancer*, London: Routledge

Stiefel, F & Krenz, S (2013) 'Psychological challenges for the oncology clinician who has to break bad news' in A Surbone, M Zwitter, M Rajer & R Stiefel, Eds, *New Challenges in Communication with Cancer Patients*, Dordrecht: Springer, 51–62

Taylor, Shelley E (1983) 'Adjustment to threatening events: a theory of cognitive adaptation', *American Psychologist*, 38, 1161–1173

Timmermans, Stefan (1994) 'Dying of awareness: the theory of awareness contexts revisited', *Sociology of Health & Illness*, 16, 322–339

Titmuss, R M (1971) *The Gift Relationship: From Human Blood to Social Policy*, London: George Allen & Unwin

Wilson, Sharon & Morse, Janice M (1991) 'Living with a wife undergoing chemotherapy', *Image: The Journal of Nursing Scholarship*, 23, 78–84

4

THE LAST WALTZ

This final chapter in *The Dance to Death* details events in the last 144 days, approximately five months of the Illness Period. There are three stories: Reviewing, Part[y]ing, and Dying. It begins with the final chemotherapy session and another CT scan.

Reviewing

The Christmas Eve news that the tumour marker is rising once again gives renewed enthusiasm for the last chemo session. However, the destructive effect on Jane's blood profile has now spread to the neutrophils, a type of white blood cell responsible for fighting infection and reducing inflammation. The clinical team are reluctant for treatment to proceed but realise its importance for Jane as revealed in an email from the oncology registrar to the consultant. At the time we were unaware of the efforts to give as much treatment as clinically possible.

> Hi – Jane is on cycle 4 of weekly Carbo/taxol and has only managed day 1 because her platelets have stagnated between 70–81. Her Ca125 has gone up this week. She is worried about the fact that she will not have had chemo [for a fortnight]. I am concerned that her Ca125 has turned up. She is keen for 1 more chemo at least next week and I thought that may be reasonable. I hope she can be treated next Thursday with a dose reduction in carbo.
>
> *(Oncology registrar email, 23 December 2011)*

Despite the gloomy realisation that the treatment is not working, there is another abdominal CT scan due before the next appointment with the oncologist. On this occasion it is at another hospital albeit in the same group, nevertheless the protocol is different. A package arrives in the post with a bottle of contrast medium and instructions, Alice in Wonderland style, to be drunk thirty minutes before attending. The hospital is in a neighbouring town necessitating an adventure to find it, the car park and the x-ray department. The difference between the two approaches for the same procedure is unclear.

> Jane duly drank the [contrast medium] and it was only about half a pint, nothing like as much as she normally had to drink. So we found the x-ray unit and it was a much smaller place and there was no waiting room full of people trying to drink these great jugs of aniseed flavoured stuff. She didn't have to drink any more, it was all very quick and efficient. We said we didn't understand why the procedure was different. They said that was how they did it there and they didn't have a waiting area as they do at the [usual hospital] and so they couldn't have people there for an hour before with jugs of stuff. I thought, well it's much nicer this way but I think it's to do with compliance and making sure that people actually drink the stuff. Otherwise the scan was much the same and the reward was to go to our favourite garden centre for lunch and that was good.
>
> *(Interview Six, 10 September 2013)*

We are puzzled by the difference in the procedure although Jane is just glad there is less to drink and that it is over quickly. For me there is a grumbling frustration as to why, when the health care team know how ill she is, do they exacerbate her discomfort by making her drink more contrast medium than clinically necessary? In the previous chapter, when we failed to understand the temporal detail of the weekly chemotherapy cycle, I suggested that Smith's (2005) 'ruling relations' were evident. To really explore the issue of the impact of hospital procedures on patients' lives would need a separate, possibly institutional ethnographic, study. Rankin and Campbell (2009) claim that the neoliberal agenda with its emphasis on efficiency and effectiveness has led to the subordination of nurses' judgement. This subordination is manifest in the "theory-practice gap" (Rolfe, 1998: 673) where there is a crisis of confidence in professional nursing knowledge. In this situation a nurse might have realised that Jane would have difficulty accommodating a large volume of liquid and raised the issue with the radiologist who could have recommended a reduction without detriment to the efficacy of the scan. This would demonstrate a recognition by the nurse of scientific knowledge (head) regarding the scan, personal knowledge (heart) of the patient, Jane, and the nurse's experiential knowledge (hand) about such situations (Rolfe, 1998). However, the x-ray department nursing staff are focused on the efficient throughput of patients and ensuring work proceeds smoothly. The idea of personalised patient care is lost in the "contingent embodiment of the universal" (Frank, 2001: 358) where the individual needs and nuances of each patient are subordinated into a generalised operational mode.

The hospital visit is soon forgotten as we celebrate Hogmanay, gathering in the kitchen to watch the fireworks and toast the new year. I abandon my daily diary feeling it would become a painful burden to record Jane's dying. Instead Jane has a new pink diary and decides to note the best thing that happens each day. Her second entry reads "Afternoon at home knitting, listening to Parsifal. Very calm" (Jane's diary, day 202). Then it is time to take the Canadian contingent (my sister and her husband) to the airport for a difficult parting as Jane notes "Such sweet sorrow, agreed they will come back in September and we will go to Islay for my birthday" (Jane's diary, day 210). We all know it is most unlikely this promise will be kept but all is not lost, the second laparoscopy is yet to come and it is important for us all in parting, to retain the veneer of optimism.

At the next clinic appointment the lead oncologist is quite upbeat:

> I saw this lady at the outpatient clinic today. Her recently performed CT scan shows a further response to therapy. The lady's CA-125 level has essentially continued to fall throughout her treatment. The interpretation of the CA-125 levels is slightly complicated by the fact that the assays have been performed at two different hospitals but there has been a steady fall until [the previous month] (Nadir 2049) and a very small rise [in the most recent] sample (2080).
>
> The lady herself is feeling extremely well. She has lots of energy and is still climbing hills and using her exercise bike. The lady tells me she has a date for a diagnostic laparoscopy and if it appears that her disease is operable then she will proceed to surgery as a combined procedure with the Colorectal surgeons and possibly the Urologists.
>
> *(Oncologist's letter to GP, 12 January 2012)*

For some reason we have a copy of this letter and it is quite helpful. It provides some resolution to the confusion regarding the CA-125 results and it reminds us of the possibility that any surgical procedure is likely to result in bowel resection and the need for a stoma. However, Jane finds the idea of a colostomy abhorrent despite my efforts to reassure her that we will deal with whatever happens. It is as if the disease being hidden deep inside her permitted innocent ignorance. A visible and artificial change to her body by the appearance of a 'poo bag' is beyond contemplation. But she is encouraged by her 'good report' and does not want to dwell on the negative aspects of surgery should it indeed prove possible. The focus was on the diagnostic laparoscopy and then all would be clear.

The preparations for the laparoscopy begin the week before the scheduled admission with a visit to the hospital for a 'pre-admission check', a chest x-ray and an ECG (electrocardiogram). On the previous occasion, at the time of diagnosis, much of the formality had been circumvented by the surgeon in his haste to get Jane into theatre. Now we have time for a minor incident during one of the pre-admission procedures:

VA: There was bit of a fuss about the ECG because when she had the ECG and then she asked if she could have a copy of the print-out cos it's all just done now as single sheet with all twelve leads on and the technician was very uppity and said no, she couldn't. Was she a cardiologist and Jane said no, she wasn't a cardiologist but it was a tracing of her heart so she would quite like to have one. I was interested because I used to do twelve lead ECGs and could interpret them. Whilst I knew there was nothing wrong with her heart, it somehow seemed important to have a tracing of her heart rhythm. But the technician wouldn't let us have it and Jane was quite annoyed about it because there are these very misunderstood rules about what people can have and what they can't have. Certainly if you ask doctors they will give you copies of things but if you ask technicians then they won't.

INTERVIEWER: So she liked having this information?

VA: Oh yes, hugely because of her father being a lab technician. I suppose it was about understanding the part of her that was ill, the things that were wrong with her body, her way of dealing with that was to understand the mechanics of it so she wanted to see things or to understand things to a point.

(Interview Seven, 8 October 2013)

It is not a legal right for an individual to see their own health record[1] and there are layers of legislation to protect both patient confidentiality and health care professionals, the most pertinent being the Data Protection Act (1998).[2] However, attitudes towards patients having easy access to their health records have started to change. In the information era of the twenty-first century there is perhaps a not unreasonable assumption that if data exists about us as individuals, we have a right not only to see that data but also for errors to be rectified. The UK devolved NHS has taken different approaches and in England since 2015 patients have online access to their primary health records[3] (Davies, 2012). In contrast the approach in Scotland could be perceived as more cautious but there is a commitment in the Scottish Government's eHealth Strategy to support people to 'manage their own health and wellbeing' (Scottish Government, 2012). Later in the same policy document a bolder statement is made, "eHealth could contribute to a radical transformation in the delivery of health and social care services in Scotland through enabling people to access and interact with their health records electronically".

Initially such services have been piloted through the management of long term health conditions such as diabetes with the integration of local authority citizen services. The vision for Scotland by 2017 is a common set of IT services with people being enabled to communicate with the health service through a medium of their own choosing. While these government initiatives are to be welcomed, there are others driven by individuals to integrate the data they gather about themselves through fitness and health monitoring programmes to be incorporated into their personal health record. Apple have now included their Health app as standard in their mobile devices (iPads and iPhones). Other tablet and smartphone manufacturers have produced similar applications. Nevertheless, this 'mobile health revolution' comes with its own health warnings as there is little evidence of the effectiveness of such apps and users are increasingly bewildered by the myriad offerings (Eng & Lee, 2013).

The value of integrated electronic health records remains some way from its true potential. As people access health services through many different agencies and services the reality of a single unified health record seems increasingly unlikely. While a relatively small country like Scotland may achieve some success with such provision, larger more complex countries such as England further lessen the reality. It has been suggested that it may be more practical and achievable to turn the issue on its head and to think in terms of a personal (not patient) health record owned and managed by the individual and held electronically (Al-Ubaydli, 2012). This record moves with the person and can be integrated with both conventional health care services and personal health monitoring data. However, giving easy access to professional health records will require not just a change in the mindsets of health care workers but a transition period of one or two years. This would allow clinicians to change the way they write up their notes and to use more accessible language. An embargo on retrospective access to existing records would also be needed to protect clinicians from records created under different rules (Al-Ubaydli, 2012). Returning to Jane's experience of having an ECG, she was sufficiently irritated to write soon after:

> I had an ECG this morning, as part of a set of routine checks prior to a scheduled admission to hospital next week for a diagnostic procedure. I've not had an ECG before, and was of course interested in the process and equipment, and particularly in the result which came out of the side of the machine on a beautifully printed sheet of figures and lines.
>
> 'Could I have a copy please?' I asked the girl who had stuck the electrodes on my chest and legs and turned on the machine. 'No you can't', she said, 'we don't give them out'. 'Why not?' I asked. 'Because of confidentiality', she said. 'But it's my heart', I said, uncomprehending. 'Well it's fine', she said. 'Are you a cardiographer?' 'No, I just have an interest in the beatings of my heart', I answered, but she had left the room.
>
> I do understand that most patients are probably only interested in the 'it's fine' bit and do not care about the squiggles on the bit of paper that represent electrical activity in the heart. Probably the said squiggles would not have meant very much to me anyway. But they were my squiggles.
>
> For the most part, the health professionals I have come across over the past few months (and there have been many) have been really informative as well as caring. However, there have been occasions when a consultant has been looking at a screen or a report and telling me things I am not really taking in, when a copy of the report would really help me to understand what is going on. I've never actually seen any of the many CT scans that have been taken of my chest and pelvis, and I'm curious. I appreciate that this is not what everyone would want, and the 'it's fine' bit is the crucial point of any diagnosis, but I get quite vexed when it feels like people are holding information about me that they are not conveying, for whatever reason. And information about me should surely not be withheld from me because of 'confidentiality' (especially

if that's being used as an excuse for 'you are not qualified to understand this information' or a euphemism for 'you might panic if you did').

I also feel that this 'doctor knows best' attitude does not really serve the national health service. Instead, it perpetuates the sense of a national illness-treating service. To be truly healthy, we need to be interested in our own well-being, engaged in the identification of the problem and implementation of the solution, and empowered to do all we can to support our own recovery. This applies whether we are talking about cancer or a throat infection. I like to know, or at least to have the option of deciding whether I want to know or not. But at any rate, my heart is just fine thanks.

(Blog post 'Power, Control & Responsibility', 24 January 2012)

This incident may seem to be rather trivial for someone with advanced cancer but Jane's own account does reveal both a need for information specific to her (as opposed to general pamphlets about ovarian cancer) and her realisation that she did not always 'hear' what was being said to her in consultations. Between our two recollections of an encounter with a clinician, we usually managed to reconstruct a reasonably coherent and accurate version of what had been said, but it would have been much easier if there had been something for reference such as a printout of a report. On occasions we did have copies of certain documents and I remember that both the original discharge letter with its explicitly detailed provisional diagnosis and the later CT scan report given by the surgeon, were highly prized and much read.

As an educator I have come to understand this need for precise information in pedagogical terms. Clinicians continue to divulge information in a didactic or instructional manner – they tell the patient what they believe is necessary, sparing actual and temporal detail in case it should cause anxiety. The patient as static recipient of the information willingly adopts the subordinate role of obedient pupil 'listening' to what is said while not actually 'hearing'. Sometimes props such as simplified diagrams are used to explain specific details of an individual case. However, as the British public generally have a very poor understanding of basic anatomy including those with medical conditions (Weinman et al., 2009), curious and stylised pictures such as those in practical guides to understanding cancer as produced by Macmillan[4] are likely to be of little use. If a patient as an informal learner, already befuddled with misinformation or erroneous ideas, is then told something awful about their inner workings, it is unsurprising if they fail to grasp what has been said. It can be all too easy for health professionals to hide behind a fear of causing unnecessary anxiety if patients are offered more explicit and detailed information about their condition.

Jane's point was about choice, the right to have the information and in a portable form, not simply just the story as told in the consultation. In a doctoral study of awareness context theory in an oncology setting, Furber (2010) ignores the pedagogical needs of the patient in understanding their diagnosis (Friberg et al., 2007). While she emphasises the educational needs of doctors as they learn to give difficult news and information to patients, she does not address the steep learning curve presented to the vast majority of patients at diagnosis. She proposes that better education and support for doctors will facilitate improvements in patient communication, which is a rather one-sided solution to a two-way process. The nature of inter-professional dialogue has been explored by Hovey and Craig (2011), who are concerned to distinguish between learning *with, from, and about* (their italics) seeing each encounter as a learning relationship with "a unique opportunity to learn inter-professionally among unique individuals" (Hovey & Craig, 2011: 267). If this awareness was extended to the formal interactions between the doctor and the patient in clinical settings, there might be some potential for enhancing patient understanding of their condition.

Our focus for the past few weeks has been on the laparoscopy which the oncologist wants done to assess the progress of the treatment. This is in addition to the CT scans and the CA-125 results which seemed to indicate there was little reduction in the size and extent of the tumour. Jane attends the same unit she was in six months previously as an emergency but this time it is relatively calm and certainly planned. The most memorable part of the episode for me, is Jane being prepared for and then wheeled away in her bed to the operating theatre.

INTERVIEWER: The next entry [in the storyboard] is the actual diagnostic laparoscopy and what was the hope for Jane from this?

VA: We had to be there for eight o'clock in the morning and she was to wait in one of the single rooms. Quite a fuss was made by the staff about this room and it certainly looked a little bit different because it had lots more lights and wood panelling at the end. It was apparently the room that had been prepared for the former prime minister's wife to be delivered of a baby. Jane was very taken with this room and it went along with treating her royally, so we had a laugh about that. Then the surgeon came bouncing in to consent her for the laparoscopy and he said that there was a possibility that he would have more time on the list and he might as well consent her for the whole thing. So we said what did he mean? If he thought that he could resect the tumour then he would do that so she was consented not just for the diagnostic laparoscopy but for the total hysterectomy and everything else.

So there was this overwhelming situation of thinking for some reason he was suddenly going to be able to do something and you get caught up in that. They eventually came to take her to theatre and I can still see her clearly, sitting up in bed with this huge grin on her face, she can't see because they've taken her glasses but she thinks they're going to fix her. I felt as though I'd been stabbed because I knew they couldn't fix her and yet there's that sliver that maybe, just maybe he's going to go in there and think 'after all I can get this out'. We knew he was just capitalising on the fact that he might have some theatre time so if he felt like having a fiddle, he could. But that cut right across all of the stuff that had been said previously about if they are going to do something it's going to need, at the very least, the bowel specialists but probably the urologists as well. Suddenly, he's a magician, he can do the whole thing. It was just awful, absolutely awful.

INTERVIEWER: Did you and Jane have time to talk about that before she went away?

VA: A wee bit, I just remember saying you know the chances are very slim, it's not likely, and if they do do something you're going to wake up with other bits attached to you and stuff and she knew all that. But it's like somebody offers you a lottery ticket and says that there's a one in ten chance of [it] coming up. This was a one in a million, the odds were appalling but I suppose from her point of view, going to theatre with a sense of elation was quite nice and that's certainly how she looked. For me it was just another gut-wrenching session and then a few hours of worrying about what was going on. I thought at the time that whilst I understood he was doing it for the best of intentions, it was actually quite a cruel thing to do and that maybe we should have just said no, go away, stop it. But then what was the point of doing the diagnostic laparoscopy if he couldn't, if there wasn't some chance that something could be done.

INTERVIEWER: I hear how strongly you feel about that. Afterwards did Jane feel that that was a cruel thing, did she have a sense of that, do you think?

VA: She certainly felt that it was yet another go on the roller-coaster that we didn't like being on; there had been quite a few episodes where your hopes are raised and then dashed by equal heights and depths and it was quite a hard one.

(*Interview Seven, 8 October 2013*)

There is no radical surgery and the reality of what the surgeon actually saw through the laparoscope is clear from the operation note:

> Unable to fully visualise pelvic organs, partially mobile uterus but fixed left ovary. Utero-vesical peritoneum obliterated by disease. Mod amount of ascites. Widespread miliary disease in pelvis, pelvic organs stuck. Tumour in omentum, Port site mets palpable. Not surgically ressectable. Diaphragms covered, porta hepatis involved.
>
> (*Hospital Operation Note, 1 February 2012*)

The operation note is almost unchanged from the original at the time of diagnosis (210 days earlier):

> Unable to visualise pelvic organs, fixed pelvis. Utero-vesical peritoneum obliterated by disease. Large amount of ascites. Widespread miliary disease in pelvis, pelvic organs stuck. Tumour in omentum. Not surgically ressectable. Diaphragms covered, porta hepatis involved.
>
> (*Hospital Operation Note, 6 July 2011*)

The main difference now is that there is tumour growth at the port site of the previous laparoscopy (the small hole made by the surgeon in the abdominal wall to permit the insertion of the laparoscope). Once Jane has recovered from the anaesthetic, the surgeon comes to see us and we have a candid discussion about his findings. He suggests that if the oncologist has some magic chemotherapy and can get the tumour marker below 1,000 then he might be able to do something. He seems so desperate to try that he cannot bring himself to say to us what is stated in the operation notes on both occasions: the tumour cannot be removed by surgery. Jane notes in her diary "Had diagnostic lap – didn't need to stay overnight. Came home for macaroni cheese & choc ice & cuddles" (Jane's diary, 1 February 2012).

It is during this time that my sister sends an email with a picture of herself holding her print *Les Deux Solitudes* which appears on the front cover of this book. We were familiar with the single image of the dancing woman having had an earlier version of the print hanging on the wall at home for many years. But this print with the woman moving through light and dark, in shadow and shade, seemed to capture something about our situation. In my reply to her email, I comment on the progress regarding an appointment for a review with the oncologist at the outpatient clinic:

> No news here yet – Jane phoned yesterday to be told it might be next week and there was no urgency if she was feeling fine! Well yes she is but we don't want to lose the momentum if there's still a chance they can operate.
>
> *(Personal email, 7 February 2012).*

We seem to be clinging to "the magical power of treatment" (The, 2002: 128) and the surgeon's idea that the oncologist has some magic chemo.

INTERVIEWER: And you talk about not losing the momentum, what was that momentum?
VA: Just the momentum of thinking something was going to happen, keeping Jane's strength and spirits up, trying to maintain her nutritional state, trying to maintain her level of fitness if she was going to have something done. Part of what had carried her through chemo was that she was working towards something that was going to have some sense of success in terms of treatment. That door was closing, but the surgeon had left it ajar and it was up to the oncologist to close it and so we needed to know. Was he closing the door, was that it or should we keep on trying.

(Interview Seven, 8 October 2013)

In due course, we attend the oncology clinic, a fortnight after the laparoscopy. The biopsies taken during the laparoscopy confirm Jane has 'metastatic high grade serous ovarian carcinoma' and that her CA-125 has started to rise. We have an honest discussion with the oncologist which he alludes to in his letter to the GP:

> In terms of symptoms she describes more discomfort/twinges over the last couple of weeks but these only last for seconds. She also feels slightly more

distended and has noticed masses around her port sites. We had a discussion today regarding the situation. I felt that a few weeks off chemotherapy would benefit the lady even though her disease is clearly slowly progressing. She knows that the disease is incurable and feels that quality of life is an important issue for her.

(Oncologist's letter to GP, 15 February 2012)

The final sentence is evidence of Jane's prognostic awareness (Innes & Payne, 2009) and what matters to her. Some other less toxic (than chemotherapy) treatment options are mooted but their availability is dependent on further genetic tests. In her diary she writes "Hamamelis bright yellow against blue sky in the Botanics this afternoon" (Jane's diary, day 246). She does not dwell on what cannot be fixed or changed, choosing to focus on the bright, the beautiful, and optimistically reflected the following day:

My lovely oncologist, who, lovely as he is, is not able to offer a ready solution to my current problem. The tumour is too large, and too widespread, for surgery to be an option (certainly not at present, and probably not at all). Additional chemotherapy is unlikely to have any positive effect on the malignancy at present either. [He] is investigating whether my tumour might respond to Tamoxifen, which is used primarily to treat breast cancer, and also my eligibility (in pathological terms) for a new gene-based drug trial. In the meantime, we have lots of trips and treats planned. We're getting through the initial list of 'things to do in Edinburgh', but there are plenty more to keep us amused. Family and friends in the West continue to offer love and support. Team Canada is onside, and reconciled (we hope) to a continuing schedule of away-only fixtures. We'll get cycling in the bulbfields this Spring. Everything is going to be alright.

(Blog Post, 'Everything is Going to be Alright', 16 February 2012)

We spend the next fortnight going for long walks, Jane enthused and exhilarated with the effort. Then back to the outpatient clinic hoping to hear there are other treatment options. The oncologist is kind but does not prevaricate. There is a one in ten chance a particular genetic test will suggest a new biological agent can be tried, but the reality is there are no more treatment options. We raise the possibility of a few days holiday in the Dutch bulb fields; he looks aghast and mutters that we would need to be 'maxed out on insurance'. We hear this and abandon such ideas. The situation is clear in his letter to the GP:

I saw this lady at the out-patient clinic. She was describing increased abdominal distension and dyspnoea which was getting worse on a daily basis. She also describes early satiety. Physical examination today revealed tense ascites with obvious shifting dullness. I discussed the fact that the lady's ascites had already recurred and we [will arrange] for the lady to be admitted for drainage of ascites.

We discussed the fact that unfortunately future therapeutic options would be limited (the rate of progression of the lady's disease following what is essentially our best chemotherapy regimen makes me fairly pessimistic about the chance of eliciting a response to other cytotoxic agents). The lady understood this discussion. If she did push for a trial of another agent then I could certainly discuss this with her.

(Oncologist's letter to GP, 29 February 2012)

The treatment door is firmly closed, this is now the turn to face death. Jane is swelling and ageing fast. Fluid has accumulated in her abdomen to such an extent that the most basic of life functions, breathing and eating, are impeded by the pressure and volume. Her movement is restricted by the weight and girth of her distended belly. Her legs have swollen as the fluid finds other places to fill. In her diary she writes "Bob and Aggie [our cats] on either side of me on the couch, tranquil, beneficent, guarding" (Jane's diary, day 258). She is neither down nor out. In this stark reality, living must now make way for dying. The first story in this chapter has described the shift from the possibilities of surgery and further treatment to rapid decline as the advancing disease continues.

Part[y]ing

In this penultimate story I describe Jane's acceptance of her situation. A stream of family and friends from near and far pay homage at her court; it is a time of partying and parting. But first there is the matter of draining the excess fluid from her abdomen as promised by the oncologist at the clinic visit. I email my sister the following day:

Here things are not quite so good. We went to the clinic and the results weren't back for the tamoxifen and we thought Jane would probably have to have some of the excess fluid, which has been accumulating over the last few weeks, drained off. Sure enough we were back at the [hospital] for 9am yesterday morning for an ultrasound and then in [the day unit] until 4.30 after the insertion of a drain and 2.6 litres being drained. Jane feels the better of it but still has a fairly swollen belly. So the treatment worked for a wee while but the tumour is back on the march and there's not much more the NHS can do apart from dealing with symptoms. But we're persevering with the herbal things and the sunny disposition although sometimes the sky gets a wee bit grey and there's some rain.

(Personal email, 2 March 2012)

The long and tedious procedure takes all day but I turn it into an outing complete with a picnic basket of provisions. Jane is admitted to the day unit by a hyper-efficient clinical nurse specialist (I am so jealous) and then sent for an ultrasound for 'x to mark the spot'. For the actual insertion of the drain, I am in my element: a surgical procedure. Jane is curious and interested. I provide a continuous commentary of all that is being done; the staff stoically get on with their work. I try not to be irritating but feel I must protect Jane from all but the absolutely necessary. Once the tube is in place, drainage proceeds cautiously for fear of causing shock by removing too much fluid at once (Stephenson & Gilbert, 2002). There is turning from side to side, walking about and generally trying to get as much fluid out and into the drainage bag. Finally, the tube runs dry and we can go home. Jane makes no mention in her diary but does note "Mum's come through to stay for a couple of days – opportunity for a candid chat about options and prognosis" (Jane's diary, day 261). Two days later she writes "Long talk with Mum this morning really cathartic for us both. Walk in sunshine this afternoon, glad to be alive" (Jane's diary, 3 March 2012).

The relief from the ascites drainage is short-lived as Jane has now developed low back pain, or at least it has started to bother her more than previously. We decide she should start taking regular analgesics. I had done some online research about palliative care, as much to find out about current practice, and came across the idea of an analgesic pathway. This concept was introduced by the World Health Organization (WHO, 1990, 2004) as an analgesic ladder with three steps or rungs of increasingly strong analgesic medication. Level one is non-opioid drugs such as ibuprofen and paracetamol which are widely available to the general public. The second stage introduces a mild opioid, codeine which is also available without prescription. Finally, level three introduces opiates which are only available on prescription and in various forms ranging from an oral linctus, through slow-release tablets to injections. The drugs at each stage all have potential side effects such as gastric irritation. Opiates especially can cause severe constipation and initially vomiting necessitating counter-measures such as laxatives and anti-emetics. Before Jane has time to develop any real side-effects of the regular analgesic regime, we visit the GP for a review. The doctor makes an entry in the online records system which can then be accessed by all members of the primary health care team:

> Consultation: Advancing ovarian Ca. Increasing ascites. Last drained 6 days ago. Increasing already. Some low back pain particularly at night. Partner and her believe it is muscular in nature. Keen to try diazepam. Taking regular paracetamol and ibuprofen for pain relief. Given oramorph PRN and diazepam. Agree to referral to Marie Curie.
>
> *(Primary health care record, 7 March 2012)*

This is it, the shift to palliation, the boundary transition between life and death (Froggatt, 1997). The GP does not prevaricate about the analgesia; Jane needs the strong stuff. I am relieved but know this news for what it is, the slow walk towards death within the next few months, hopefully not weeks. Referral to the community nurses and the palliative care service provided by Marie Curie are mentioned as necessary next steps. We express our gratitude and acceptance of such support. Unsurprisingly although the morphine provides excellent pain relief, it also makes

Jane very sick, a symptom that is to be a major feature of her remaining months. I email my sister following the visit to the GP:

> Here things are not great as her majesty is somewhat indisposed with back pain and today has been taking the order of the barf. We're not sure if this is because of pressure on the stomach or a change in analgesics (morphine's lovely stuff but it can sometimes be barfy). Anyway I'm sure a good night's sleep and a quiet day will be restorative. We had hoped to go up to Abriachan tomorrow to collect plants but I'm drawing the line at buckets in the car. Her majesty will probably also be needing drained again early next week so nothing but fun for us. Please try not to worry about us, we're fine and it's all ok.
>
> *(Personal email, 8 March 2012)*

Somehow it is much easier for me to write in euphemistic language and make a joke of the situation while being open and honest. Part of my coping mechanism is resorting to black or gallows humour, a throwback to when I worked in A & E. While this may seem inappropriate, it has been suggested it is a way of moving forward, from the horrific accident victim to the next patient (Watson, 2011). A systematic review of the use of humour by nurses found it a poorly researched area and suggested nurses should be circumspect in its use but aware of its value to release tension (McCreaddie & Wiggins, 2008). More positively, Smyth (2011) believes laughter has a place in palliative care. While I write with euphemistic humour, Jane takes a more direct approach when writing to her scientific cousin:

> You may have gathered the news on the health front is not great. There's still a chance of a couple of drug trials but basically the forward plan is to 'keep me comfortable' for as long as possible. This includes day hospitalisation to insert a tube to drain off some of the fluid that gathers in my belly from time to time, which is a bit unpleasant but not as ghastly as it might sound. Otherwise we are just staying calm. Mum came through for a couple of days last week which was lovely, and a good opportunity for a long heart-to-heart. Life is too short to leave things unsaid!
>
> *(Personal email, 7 March 2012)*

Our humour and fortitude are severely tested at the weekend as the ascites has gathered again causing pain and pressure:

> There was an awful, awful weekend when I thought she was going to burst. She was in considerable discomfort with it and very nauseated. The real problem was that the day unit only operates Monday to Friday so she couldn't go to have the ascites drained out with those hours. I was quite frustrated because when we'd gone for the initial drain they'd talked about how there was a new permanent drain. So I said well, can't we just do that then instead of keep putting Jane through this. But there's a protocol and there's a big cost

implication because the drainage bottles cost £40 so special permission had to be granted. So we had this dreadful weekend where she just had swollen right up massively and in a lot of pain until we eventually got to the Monday and she could go in to have it drained.

(Interview Eight, 15 October 2013)

This account gives some sense of the grim reality of advanced ovarian cancer 'an awful, awful weekend' and my frustration at the apparent vagaries of the health service where 'special permission had to be granted'. It is hard to watch the pain and intolerable discomfort of the ascites whilst feeling powerless to do anything. Perhaps more effort should have been made for Jane to be admitted to hospital where, even at the weekend, the drainage procedure could have been performed. However, she is seen by various community doctors, none of whom propose hospitalisation as an option; this was after all, a palliative situation. By Monday almost ten litres of ascites has accumulated; this was the great drainage. Three days later Jane notes the beneficial effect "Had sticky rice and smoked cod for tea and I was really hungry" (Jane's diary, day 276). During the admission for the paracentesis, Jane is told that the result of the oestrogen receptor test indicated Tamoxifen (a hormone antagonist) might be beneficial. The potential efficacy of hormone therapies that disrupt ovarian tumour growth has been known for many years (Hatch et al., 1991) and more precise therapies are becoming available (Smyth et al., 2007). For Jane, treatment is started:

As the lady's primary tumour has an ER histoscore of 260 the aims and toxicities of Tamoxifen therapy were discussed with her. It was explained that Tamoxifen is licensed for breast carcinoma but not for ovarian carcinoma although some patients do benefit. In addition plans are being put in place to have a PleurX catheter inserted in order to facilitate future drainages.

(Hospital record, 13 March 2012)

The referral by the GP to the palliative care services has initiated visits from two important services, Marie Curie and the community (district) nurses. The week after the great drainage, the Marie Curie nurse visits for the first time. We have an open and frank discussion with her about what we know and understood of Jane's condition and prospects. Jane wants to die at home but realises that as her condition deteriorates this might not be practicable. A few days later the district nurse arrives with a student nurse in tow:

The district nurse came for the initial visit to ascertain the lie of the land. Jane was on the couch in the window and [the district nurse] proceeded to say a little bit about what she could do and what might need to happen. We knew exactly what was going on, Jane was going to die, that wasn't going to be too long, she might need some additional care but Jane wanted to stay at home. So [the district nurse] kind of looked about and said well yes that would be

fine but of course we'd need to bring in a hospital bed. At this point I looked at Jane and thought I'd better get the bucket and she was then very sick which startled both the district nurse and the student nurse. It wasn't entirely unexpected but I knew it was because Jane was really wound up about the prospect of bringing a hospital bed into our small flat and all of the upheaval that that would cause and the impact that that would have on us and not least our cats.
(Interview Eight, 15 October 2013)

Dying was hard enough but the prospect of it being somewhere strange, not at home (unhomelike) in her own bed, is just too much for Jane to bear. Her visceral reaction startles those present but the message seems clear. Jane is finding it difficult to press for what she wants as her strength wanes. However, the district nurse arranges for a ripple mattress to be delivered for Jane's side of the bed. Froggatt (1997) in her analysis of hospice settings and structures describes the journey from life to death as a rite of passage, when entry into hospice care marks the transition from the secular world. This is the separation from normal life (the life as known) until reincorporation after death through funerary rituals. When hospice and palliative care are provided in the person's own home, that place becomes sacred. There are rights and rituals to be respected. A ritual for us is asking people to remove their shoes on entry to the flat, although I am too fazed to ask visiting doctors. At a deeper level, I wonder if Jane's reaction to the prospect of a hospital bed is because she has recently entered a liminal or threshold state and wants to assert her right to die in her own bed, a recent acquisition. The bed has its own sacred qualities, handmade for us in walnut, a wood associated with healing and inner peace.

Jane continues discussions with her family "Talked to [sisters and mother] about lack of any funeral. All ok I think" (Jane's diary, day 278). Then two days later "I have written 'what you mean to me' emails to [sisters and cousins]. Had long talk with [cousins]. Feeling very very warm and loved" (Jane's diary, day 280). She also has a discussion with my sister "Didn't just talk about sickness and death but mostly did. Now it's all said we can all get on with the rather splendid business of living" (Jane's diary, day 283). Reflecting on this time now, it seems as if the great draining both energised Jane and galvanised her into addressing family matters. She realised her life was diminishing but wanted to act on her feelings while she could. The relief of the great drainage is more temporary than we hoped, as I tell my sister:

Her majesty has turned into Mme Creosote[5] and is fine as long as she doesn't have a wafer thin mint or any other solid food. But she is doing very well on full strength Ovaltine and special leek & potato soup with extra milk protein. We have to persevere until next Monday when they will do the permanent drain which will makes things a lot easier. So that's some good news, it's just a bit of pain they can't do it until next week but it's a boss man that has to supervise and he's very busy (obviously no one has told him it's for royalty).
(Personal email, 21 March 2012)

The management of malignant[6] ascites has exercised the health profession for many years (Stephenson & Gilbert, 2002). The most common cause of fluid accumulating in the abdomen is due to cirrhosis but 20 per cent of ascites are non-hepatic in origin (Stanojević et al., 2004). Consequently until recently the evidence for appropriate treatment protocols was based on best practice in the context of liver disease and not malignancy, despite the very different pathology (Stephenson & Gilbert, 2002). Essentially there are two ways in which accumulated excess fluid might be removed from the abdomen, either by drug therapy or by manual drainage. There was sufficient concern within the gynaecological oncology community for Macdonald et al. (2006) to conduct a survey of clinical staff on the management of ascites in ovarian cancer. They found considerable variation between both clinical speciality – gynaecologists tended to use more interventions than physicians (oncologists and palliative consultants) – and between hospital settings, where diuretics were preferred to paracentesis in palliative centres. The limited efficacy of diuretics was noted by Mercadante et al. (2008) who favoured a permanent peritoneal catheter to facilitate home drainage and reduce the symptom burden. However, the authors also noted that at the time no catheter designed for peritoneal use existed and their solution was therefore unlicensed. This combined with the lack of a standardised protocol for the palliative treatment of malignant ascites prompted Fleming et al. (2009) to conduct a systematic review and recommend a permanent solution for repeated paracenteses.

The symptoms experienced by women with ovarian malignant ascites are distressing and troublesome. In addition to the tense abdominal pressure and distension, patients may also experience nausea, vomiting, early satiety, shortness of breath, swollen legs and reduced mobility (Tapping et al., 2012). Unfortunately these symptoms also tend to occur in the last weeks and months of life making repeated hospital attendance and admissions an unwanted burden at a difficult time for both the woman and her family. Having established, as outlined in the studies cited above, the preference and efficacy of drainage over drug therapy, the need for a more permanent solution was proposed which involved the insertion of an in-dwelling plastic catheter into the abdominal cavity. The internal tubing is held in place by a fifteen centimetre section being tunnelled subcutaneously and then sutured in place. Vacuum drainage bottles are then used to suck the fluid out by negative pressure. Drainage can be done daily on the basis that a little more often is preferable to the accumulation of many litres of ascitic fluid (Tapping et al., 2012). This PleurX peritoneal drainage system has now been approved by NICE for use in England (Kmietowicz, 2012).

Other research has proposed novel drug therapies that exploit particular mechanisms in the pathophysiology of malignant ascites. For example in the healthy body there is a natural balance in the vascular environment for the maintenance of blood cells through angiogenesis, the process for the development of new blood vessels. However, in the diseased body this balance becomes disrupted as the formation of new blood vessels is demanded by the growing tumour. Vascular endothelial growth factor (VEGF) has been identified as being essential for both tumour growth and the formation of ascites, but it can be inhibited by the antibodies bevacizumab or catumaxomab (Eskander & Tewari, 2012). It is hoped that further advances in the understanding of the pathophysiology of ovarian cancer ascites and the molecular features of the disease will lead to more precise and effective treatments in the near future (Kipps et al., 2013). This optimism is tempered by the need for larger scale trials to determine both the efficacy of symptom relief and overall survival (Smolle et al., 2014).

Finally the day arrives for the insertion of the permanent drain. Jane attends the day unit and hopes to be home by evening. However, her blood biochemistry has become disrupted, another common effect of malignant ascites. As the ascitic fluid has a high protein concentration, the direction of fluid travel across the peritoneal membrane is switched so that fluid flows into as opposed to out of, the abdomen (Kipps et al., 2013). This haemodynamic mechanism was first described by the British physiologist Ernest Starling (1896), a historical point that would have fascinated Jane. The lead oncologist is on holiday and the duty registrar decides to actively treat the chemical imbalance. Had Jane's high potassium level not been treated she could have developed an arrhythmia causing her heart to stop beating. It would have been a quick and relatively painless way to die but she was not quite ready to leave (Copp, 1998).

The actual procedure for the insertion of the PleurX drain is recorded in both the discharge letter and the radiology report as being 'uneventful'. However, our experience does not concur with these observations. I am allowed to go into the x-ray theatre and stay with Jane throughout. I play my former-ward-sister-at-the-hospital card, and provided I change into scrubs, the staff are most accommodating. As Jane is pushed in a wheelchair into the theatre suite, the staff nurse acknowledges her as 'Mrs Plenderleith'. I immediately react by saying she is not 'missus' but 'doctor'. This proves to be a welcome distraction for Jane as she is then able to explain she is not a medical doctor and outlines her PhD. When I return from the changing room, she is deep in conversation with the staff nurse on the finer points of the philosophy of Moses Mendelssohn,[7] an indication that eighteenth-century German philosophy is never far from her mind. With some difficulty she manages to get onto the rigid, narrow x-ray theatre table and is asked to 'lie back'. I intervene explaining she cannot lie flat, if she does she will vomit. Jane paled, the staff insisted and she throws up, causing commotion and embarrassment. She then has to stay in hospital until her blood biochemistry stabilises. She ignores the unpleasantness and writes instead "Spent night in [hospital] – they were helping me to feel better" (Jane's pink diary, day 286).

As the PleurX drain is a new device, the manufacturer's representative comes to provide training for the hospital staff. I am allowed to participate in the training so I can manage the drain once Jane is home. The district nurse visits the day after Jane's discharge to inspect the drain and see it in operation as it is also new in the community.

> There was quite a lot of blood coming off that I'm a bit concerned about. So she did a full blood count and the results went to the hospital and they saw

that [Jane's] haemoglobin had fallen to 77.[8] So she was re-admitted and transfused with three units of packed cells but why was she bleeding? I felt sure that they had dislodged some tumour from the inside of her abdominal wall when the trocar was used to make to a hole.

(Interview Nine, 22 October 2013)

Repeated abdominal paracentesis has the potential risk of both bleeding and infection (Fleming et al., 2009); one of the cited advantages of the PleurX system is that it reduces these risks (Tapping et al., 2012). My recollection in the interview extract does offer an explanation and also alludes to my frustration when I noticed the drained fluid was heavily blood-stained. When I ask how we are to dispose of the drainage bottles I am told to empty them down the toilet and then put the bottle in the general waste. It seems there is no provision in the community for the environmentally conscious disposal of medical waste nor any great concern either. We comment to each other how quickly we have pushed aside long held beliefs and behaviours in the wake of Jane's declining health and increasing care needs. Jane makes no comment on this episode and instead writes about the food treats she is now able to enjoy. First, "Had to stay in. [Veronica] came back from Waitrose with choice food for palliative care – smoked salmon bruschetta and chocolate ice cream" (Jane's diary, day 289) and then "avocado splosh and a puzzle book to keep me busy. Fantastic view of the Edinburgh skyline from my window" (Jane's diary, day 290). The hospital discharge letter summarises events:

> Jane was admitted as an emergency from home with increasing SOB [shortness of breath] and lethargy, bloods taken by your district nursing team confirmed that Jane was anaemic. She was transfused 3 units of RBC [red blood cells], commenced on tranexamic acid and her high potassium was treated with insulin/dextrose during this admission. Jane had a CT scan which showed no active bleeding and the pleurX catheter in a satisfactory position, it did however confirm disease progression. [The oncologist] after discussion with Jane have [sic] agreed that no further bloods should be checked, the aim of treatment being symptom control with community palliative care input.
>
> *(Hospital discharge letter, 2 April 2012)*

When the lead oncologist comes to review Jane on Monday morning, she asks him a straight question, 'How much longer do you think I have?' and receives a straight answer 'a number of weeks'. Her version in a blog post omits this temporal information and gives a different interpretation:

> Meanwhile, I've been a bit poorly. Without going into too much detail, the fluid gathering in my abdomen was making eating and drinking increasingly problematic. Draining the fluid while maintaining some kind of blood chemistry balance proved something of a challenge for the NHS staff at the [hospital]

(for whom I have nothing but thanks and praise). I now have a permanent drain fitted which makes 'little and often' drainage possible. [The oncologist] came back from leave on Monday and decreed, with which [we] wholeheartedly concur, that no further heroic chemical balance exploits should be attempted, that I should be allowed to come home to my own comforts. District nurses and Marie Curie are there to help when we need them, and [Veronica is] able to drain as much or as little as we think appropriate. Even more to the point, it keeps me hungry, or peckish at least! It's official, I can eat whatever I like. Sometimes my requests are reasonably adult (I want sushi), others amusingly childish (chips, cola, chocolate ice cream). I can spend much of the afternoon deciding whether I'd rather have my hot smoked salmon peppered or honeyed, and basil or chives in my avocado salsa (with chips of course). Curiously enough, I am having a rather lovely time :)

(Blog post, 'Catching Up', 31 March 2012)

Jane's demeanour following the ascitic draining and blood replenishment give the impression of catharsis; she is energised, almost renewed. Her life is reduced to minuscule, intense and exquisite moments that she relishes and savours. These range from the food she eats through excursions out, to the many visitors who journey to see her from near and far. In this invigorated state Jane writes about her impending demise:

An archaeologist on Orkney once explained to me that nothing helps anthropologists to understand a historical civilisation and society better than its practices and traditions for dealing with its dead. Burial places, rites and rituals, accompanying objects, carvings, gravestones, mummification, ceremonial pyres, cremation, urns and ash disposal – all have something to say about how societies respect their dead. Mostly they are also expressing some kind of appreciation for the life lived. But more importantly, these funerary rites generally reflect the way a civilisation thinks its dead should be prepared and furnished for some kind of transference to another world.

Many years ago, long before my cancer diagnosis, we made the decision, and the arrangements, to donate our bodies to medical science. All usable organs were to be transferred to appropriate donors, and the rest sent to the Anatomy Department of [a university]. They won't want my organs now, but apparently there is still interest in receiving the body. So there isn't going to be any funeral for me – no body, no coffin, no service, no cremation.

I was brought up as a Christian in the Church of Scotland in Glasgow. I've always been grateful for my Sunday School grounding in the stories and imagery of the Bible, which proved essential background knowledge for an appreciation of the literature and culture of the Western Judaeo-Christian tradition (culminating, I suppose, in the subject-matter of my PhD thesis). I was a regular and enthusiastic church-attender from my teenage years. But I was finding it increasingly difficult to accept – and believe – the central tenets of the Christian faith.

When I went north to work in Inverness, I became distanced from the church, in more ways than one. I felt able to acknowledge that my 'doubts' were not a failing on my part, for which I required to do social penance. My parents taught me, by word and example and by the entirely comfortable and secure context of our upbringing, how to determine right from wrong for myself, to be kind, and fair, and understand the meaning of justice. Not being a Christian does not mean not being a good person. Not being a Christian does not mean I have not been profoundly touched by the thoughts and prayers of so many people – some known and very close to me, some complete strangers – who have been remembering me in their communion with their God these past months. It's odd that I find myself describing my position in a series of double negatives, of course. Atheism is an unpleasant word; it implies an antagonism I do not feel. If I do require a concept to describe my world-view, perhaps humanism comes closest.

Whatever you call it, it's a strong and powerful position to be in. I am reconciled to my lot, I do not rail against any external forces which have dealt me any cruel blows, I do not expect any miracles. I cannot in any conscience countenance a Christian funeral for myself. Nor even a humanist one. I do understand that funerals are intended for the mourners rather than the deceased. There's something I find entirely inappropriate about someone who never – or hardly – knew me talking about the life I lived while those I love have to sit and listen. I feel very strongly that anyone who would like to 'pay their respects' can do so – and are indeed doing so – while I am still here and able to enjoy their company and comfort. Is that terribly selfish of me? There are other ways of marking my passing than with a coffin and a crematorium. Have a party. Drink Loire fizz and fine whiskies. Eat cake and chocolate ice cream. Tell terrible jokes. Play the piano, sing very loud and out of tune. Have a laugh. It's your funerary right.

(Blog post, 'Funerary Rites', 6 April 2012)

It could be argued that by being at the centre of her own drama, Jane is maintaining her self-esteem and reducing any anxiety she has of her approaching death. This accords with the view that "In order to keep the anxiety-buffer provided by self-esteem, one must continually reaffirm one's value and one's faith in the absolute validity of one's world view" (Greenberg et al., 1986: 199). In recounting fond memories and reminiscing on her former healthy self, Jane is able to maintain her strong sense of self and the ability to cope with her situation. It has been suggested that an illusory process of looking at known facts in a particular way enables cognitive adaptation to occur (Taylor, 1983). By thinking of healthier times, Jane is able to pretend she is well and can ignore her terminal decline. However, I believe 'Funerary rites' illustrates, she was under no illusion nor particularly anxious, but she would have liked to be at the party.

Dying

This is the concluding story of *The Dance to Death* and recounts Jane's final month. From my earlier research of current palliative care guidelines, I have been privately preparing for what may need to be done. The district nurse has brought an 'anticipatory drugs pack' complete with needles, syringes and a sharps disposal box. I put them in the cocktail cupboard. The purpose of the anticipatory prescribing is for those who are dying at home to have easy access to medication without unnecessary delay. When the time comes, I am allowed to administer any of the drugs subcutaneously through a butterfly canula. There are four different drugs: an analgesic for pain or breathlessness; a sedative for anxiety or distress; an anti-secretory to help with unwanted respiratory secretions; and an antiemetic for nausea.

The metastatic tumours in Jane's abdomen are now pressing on her gastro-intestinal tract to such an extent that a complicated cocktail of drugs is prescribed in an attempt to manage the worst of the nausea and vomiting. Unfortunately but perhaps inevitably these oral drugs are not well absorbed and no longer have much effect. When the Marie Curie nurse comes for her next visit she suggests it is time for a syringe driver to continuously administer a different anti-emetic. Within hours of the decision, the district nurse arrives with a large plastic crate and sets up the syringe driver, a portable infusion pump that will last for 24 hours.

Ironically, although Jane now feels more confident that she will not vomit if she goes out, she has to carry this unwieldy contraption. However, she quickly adapts choosing a cotton bag for outings and a plastic supermarket bag for protection in the shower. All things considered, the pump boosts rather than reduces her independence. It makes a family visit to Glasgow the following day possible, even going out for lunch. Jane's is a 'paediatric' soup and pudding. We then attend a fund-raising event at her cousin's where she holds court from an armchair. It is a fortuitous opportunity for many family members who will not get to see her again. Friends continue to visit and she lists all who come in a blog posting, ending with:

> It's so lovely that people's first reaction is to come and see me. I really do feel completely surrounded by love and support. I'm calm about what's ahead, but for now, I'm thoroughly enjoying each moment of my life. Through all this, of course, [Veronica] remains an incredible tower of strength. She never stops looking out for me, listening for every breath, anything unusual, always aware of where I am, what I'm doing, what I'm eating and drinking, sorting drugs, drains and dressings. Even when she's sleeping she's still got half an ear listening for me. She's a tiny bit marvellous, to put it mildly.
>
> *(Blog post 'Friends and Family', 16 April 2012)*

I was not sure if I should include that extract about my performance as I find it embarrassing. At the time I know I wanted to be recognised as essential to Jane's well-being, but now I also recognise that again my Amazonian presence may have made it difficult for others to be involved in Jane's care.

Despite the slight reassurance afforded by the continuous drugs and the attempts to boost her nutritional status with protein milk shakes, Jane is frail and cachectic. Yet she remains keen for excursions and little adventures.

INTERVIEWER: So then, [Jane's mum] came and stayed for three nights, so how was that for Jane to have her mother there?

VA: Well she was really looking forward to [her mum] coming through to stay and the plan had been, Jane wanted to go to Alnwick to visit the poison garden at Alnwick Castle and she wanted her mum to come with us. So [her mum] had come through and I found a little hotel that we could stay in and it would only be just over an hour's drive and she was really looking forward to it. But it became quite clear to me that Jane wasn't going to manage sitting in the car for that length of time even with the syringe driver. Her symptoms were too unpredictable and I didn't want the risk of us being away somewhere and her becoming more unwell or compromised or just simply upset by being somewhere strange when she wasn't feeling up to it. And so I think I just persuaded her we should wait until things were a bit more settled and we could try again. I think [her mum] was quite relieved although she was disappointed. If Jane wanted to go on the outing then that would've been fine but she also realised that Jane wasn't up to it. So Jane's head really wanted to go but her body wouldn't let her.

INTERVIEWER: How did she, how was she then with that, that your head might want it but you can't have it?

VA: She was disappointed and I suppose it was for her, well for both of us, a real realisation that things were diminishing, things were becoming less possible. She probably didn't have much longer left. And so we would focus on what she could do. She could get up, she could sit on the couch and she could look out of the window and people could visit and that was easier for her.

INTERVIEWER: What I was picking up from what you'd written [in the storyboard] was that the outings are diminishing and it sounds like from what you're saying that the distances then become much shorter, that she's staying much closer to home.

VA: Yes, there aren't too many places she can go now and she doesn't want the hassle of having to go either, she doesn't want to have to struggle up and down the stairs. We have got a lovely view and she was very comfortable sitting on her couch and … just looking out of the window. She tires very easily. There's a lot of effort needed just to do simple things. There's no point in her being overly taxed either physically or emotionally if she doesn't need to be.

INTERVIEWER: What did she find emotionally taxing?

VA: Realising that she couldn't for example go to Alnwick, that life was shrinking. The range of things that she could do was becoming increasingly difficult. She was finding reading and writing difficult, she was finding knitting difficult. She had been a very, very active person, she'd always been busy, she'd always been doing something. She never just sat in a chair and watched the telly, she was always doing a puzzle or knitting or something else. She didn't want a life where all she could do was sit and look out of the window, if she couldn't be actively engaged in it then she was kind of loosing interest in it. But she wasn't distressed by that, she was on a fairly smooth plateau apart from the nausea and vomiting and that was quite unpleasant for her.

(Interview Ten, 29 October 2013)

Following the visit of a former work colleague, whom she had not seen for some time, Jane notes in her diary:

[Colleague] came for coffee this morning. Like it's been no time at all – instead of years – since I last saw her. Big hugs. And 'hello beautiful' is a nice way to be greeted.

(Jane's pink diary, 20 April 2012)

Jane's appearance has changed considerably since the onset of her illness. After the chemotherapy-induced alopecia, her hair has regrown into a wiry grey mop which she is no longer interested in colouring for a more youthful look. Her face is thin and gaunt, her abdomen enormous and she walks with a slow waddle. She seems to have aged thirty years in a few weeks. For someone to say with sincerity that she is beautiful is powerful and compassionate. Much as she loves to go out to parks and gardens she is now too weak and immobile to walk any distance. I hire a wheelchair, a heavy cumbersome beast, but it means I can really push her around. She takes her debility in her stride and writes "pushed around Botanics this afternoon – cold but lovely to be out in the fresh air and smell the blossom. Then we had an ice cream!" (Jane's diary, day 320). It is not many days after the start of the anti-emetic syringe driver before I have to give her an additional 'breakthrough' dose. At first it is just the odd one, not every day but the frequency gradually creeps up. A fortnight after the arrival of the syringe driver, Jane needs two or three extra doses from late evening and through the night.

I record every drug and dose I give in both the community nursing record and a spreadsheet. I do not really believe anyone is going to either question or challenge what I am doing; these are legitimately prescribed drugs. Yet I worry, wanting to give Jane the best care, still reproaching myself for not realising she was ill until it was far too late. The district nurse visits each morning to refill the syringe driver but then has to hurry away for her next visit. I want her to say we are doing okay, that everything is going to be all right. We muddle on, propping each other up through grey moments and occasional tears. Jane manages small achievements "Finished Fair Isle tea-cosy! (Also, it's 4 weeks today since 'how long' conversation with [the oncologist])" (Jane's diary, 30 April 2012).

Managing Jane's diet is also especially challenging as the disease progresses. Food, both in preparation and eating, has been one of our great shared loves.

INTERVIEWER: How did Jane deal with the kind of limited capacity she had to take in food?

VA: I suppose the thing that was difficult was that her senses, particularly smell and hearing, were enhanced by the morphine.[9] I had to be really careful with food smells of what I was eating or even indeed cat food smells because she would really notice them and they weren't particularly pleasant for her. She was taking immense and intense pleasure in very small things, so a frozen strawberry which she could suck or there were various ice creams. Ultimately it was just down to lemon sorbet.

INTERVIEWER: But there were still things that she could actually enjoy although in very small quantities?

VA: Yes, the amuse bouche had become almost microscopic, it was little intense tastes. Initially her preference was for quite savoury things. I found in one of the palliative care guidelines, it was about tempting people. Mostly they're about using really sweet things but what she wanted was something quite savoury. Mashed up egg with avocado which she found very tasty. But then, as things deteriorated eating-wise she didn't mind if things were sweeter like ice creams and sorbets, but not sickly sweet.

(Interview Eleven, 5 November 2013)

The issue of where to die remains unresolved; the spectre of the hospital bed in the living room still looms. The alternative is the hospice when the time comes. On a routine visit, the district nurse suggests Jane might benefit from a review by the palliative team of her drug therapy to try and reduce the nausea and vomiting. The experience is a defining moment for Jane.

> We have had many conversations over the past months about my final days and how best to deal with what might be ahead. I hope that will be understood as pragmatic forward planning rather than some maudlin fascination with my end. We've had many conversations about lots of other things as well. Anyway, plan A was for me to be looked after here at home. However, we were somewhat disturbed by an early conversation with the district nurse team which implied that this option was only open if we were able to accommodate a hospital bed and a commode. That was just too much to contemplate in our lovely wee flat. I couldn't really see myself lying in the window propped up in my hospital bed, waving at the passengers on the upstairs deck of each passing bus, with a commode in front of the fireplace. The commode thing is just horrendous and I am going to say no more about it. We were also slightly uneasy about how the cats would view this new sleeping arrangement, rather suspecting that they would adopt the new bed for themselves.
>
> So we came round to thinking about plan B, which was to spend my last few days (I felt, and still feel, quite strongly that I will know when this time comes, and it's not any time very soon) in the local hospice which is just ten minutes drive up the road. We went for a wee recce last week, taking

advantage of the visit for each of us to have a very pleasant relaxing massage. The grounds are lovely, especially at the moment when the cherry blossom is in full bloom. The atmosphere was calm and relaxing. One of the big arguments for hospice over home was that [Veronica] would be my partner rather than my carer at that time, and that seemed important.

I've been a bit bothered by digestive problems over the past few weeks. It's characteristic of the progression of my disease, things pressing on internal organs, and on the nervous system that generally helps things to work. I was feeling pretty awful yesterday morning when the district nurse came for her usual daily visit, and she suggested that I should admit myself to the hospice to try to get my drugs regime sorted. We concurred, got some things together, and arrived there late morning. We were shown into a room with a bed and a variety of chairs, and waited. We waited quite a long time. At about eight o'clock last night, my drugs were changed to an agreed new regime. I spent a reasonably comfortable night in the hospice. Without going into too much detail, I didn't throw up for the first time in what seems like weeks so that is a definite improvement.

However, in the course of the evening we absolutely resolved that I was getting out of the hospice today. One night was enough. The staff are kind, and well-meaning, and the hospice clearly plays a vital role in the care and support of a vast number of cancer sufferers and their families. But with the best will in the world the care is necessarily institutionalised, and dependent on staff availability rather than immediate patient needs. The nursing staff were not at all sure about letting me home, there was even talk of staying for a week. I don't have that many weeks left that I wanted to spend one there. The palliative consultant was entirely understanding and supportive of our wishes, and confident that we have the necessary wherewithal to put in place a care plan to look after me at home. Nevertheless, it did feel a little bit like a break-out, and is certainly a huge relief to be writing this from my throne by the window with my view of the hills. [Veronica] is ready and able to continue to provide entirely patient-centred care. She's there for me whenever I need whatever I want. For as long as it takes. We are back on Plan A.

(Blog post 'Breaking out of the Hospice', 2 May 2012)

Following the overnight stay in the hospice Jane now has two syringe drivers, one in each arm; the new driver contains morphine and a sedative, in the other is the anti-emetic at a much higher dose. The parting advice from the palliative care consultant, when asked if there is anything else we could or should do for Jane's comfort, is 'you have plenty of drugs in the house, so use them'. The hospice encounter highlights another aspect of Froggatt's (1998) analysis of hospice care: the sense of *communitas* exemplified by a lack of hierarchy. The palliative consultant is quick to respond to Jane's stated wishes. He phones the district nurse and dissolves her concerns regarding suitable beds for the dying and our ability to cope. Her role and attitude are framed within the secular structure of community care, where patients can be subordinated to the views and opinions of the health care professionals. By insisting that a hospital bed would be required, she is asserting her authority and status over us. In crossing the limen, preparations need to be made to care for Jane in her last days. In the sacred setting of hospice care, the patient has equal status. Curiously, the hospice itself was not quite the sacred space that Froggatt (1998) describes. What Jane does not mention is the rigid routine operated by the nursing staff, a very secular structure. Taking pills is difficult for Jane and she is accustomed to having her evening medication at a particular time. When we ask for them, we are told that the staff have started the drug round 'at the other end' so she would get hers when they are ready. So she has to wait an hour to be officially given her own medication that we have brought in with us.

Jane continues to note positive thoughts and experiences in her diary:

- Constant round of visitors & phone calls today. Exhausting but feel very loved (3 May 2012)
- [Veronica] pushed me around [the reservoir]. Sunshine, blue sky, warblers, primroses, bluebells, coconut-smelling gorse (6 May 2012)
- Went to Botanics. Loads more rhododendrons & azaleas coming into bloom, wheelchair is at optimum height for appreciating scent (8 May 2012)
- [My brother and partner] left, not saying goodbye, instead 'Skype you tomorrow' [Youngest sister] wants to cherish last memories of me on the beach at St Andrews (9 May 2012)
- [Younger sister] brought mum through this afternoon – no more visitors now. Not sorry. It's been lovely, and full of love, but I'm tired. Just me and [Veronica] now (11 May 2012)
- Dozed all day. Feel very calm and peaceful (12 May 2012)
- There's nothing quite like a frozen strawberry for reviving a droughty mouth (13 May 2012)
- Wouldn't you just die without lemon sorbet (sorry) (16 May 2012)

Friends and family offer to come and 'babysit' but I feel I cannot leave Jane with someone else. I know she just wants me to attend to everything, but I do email my sister:

> Just a wee update as I know you'll be wondering how we're doing – I was going to phone but I don't want to be a moaning minnie and mostly it's ok, just a teeny bit harder each day. Jane is getting weaker and very sleepy but manages to wake at regular intervals for lemon sorbet! The drivers seems to be alleviating the worst of her symptoms, the downside being the drowsiness. Now she's passed all her deadlines she's not making any more!
>
> *(Personal email, 16 May 2012)*

Reading this now and my excuse for not phoning, it occurs to me that I did not phone because I could not speak of what I was experiencing. The complexity of researching suffering is well understood by Frank which he describes with a precise profundity that resonates with me.

> Suffering involves experiencing yourself on the other side of life as it should be, and no thing, no material resource, can bridge that separation. Suffering is what lies beyond such help. Suffering is the unspeakable, as opposed to what can be spoken; it is what remains concealed, impossible to reveal; it remains in darkness, eluding illumination; and it is dread, beyond what is tangible even if hurtful. Suffering is loss, present or anticipated, and loss is another instance of no thing, an absence. … To suffer is to lose your grip. Suffering is expressed in myth as the wound that does not kill but cannot be healed.
> (Frank, 2001: 355)

The statement at the end of the quotation of the unhealed wound could refer to the legendary wound of Amfortas in Parsifal, as identified in the previous chapter. However, Frank does not reference Jung who recognised that the personal experience of the analyst may make them a wounded healer in relation to their patient (Samuels et al., 1986). In the thesis (Adamson, 2015) I write about having no personal experience of serious illness, but being wounded by my previous nursing experience, particularly in caring for women with advanced cancer. Now I am not so sure. At the time of the email when I did not phone my sister, it was because I would have lost my grip and there was no certainty I could have regained control. And during the doctoral research I was so very wounded yet adept at concealing the gaping wound, to acknowledge its presence would have been to fail as a nurse and as a partner.

The following day (Thursday) Jane makes her last diary entry which previously had felt too personal to share in the thesis. Now I want to include it with the realisation that the wound has healed leaving many memories but few scars, "The one good thing about today and every day is, always was, and ever will be my darling" (Jane's diary, 17 May 2012). Friday starts like most other days of the past few weeks. With great effort Jane manages to have a shower, the two syringe drivers balanced precariously on the end of the bath. Eventually she is dressed, ensconced on the couch, managing a little sorbet. Her breathing is stertorous, wherever I am in the flat, I can hear the heavy effort. In the afternoon she asks for some breakthrough morphine and then to go through to bed; she can no longer get comfortable on the couch. I help her to undress, she hugs me and says now she just wants to stay in bed. In her naked state she is, as Turner (1969: 95) describes, a 'liminal entity' without possessions to demonstrate status, property, insignia, or secular clothing. This act completes the threshold crossing to the innermost sanctum. I worry about turning her in a king size bed and pressure sores and all the other basic care drills in my head. The community nursing team produce a glide sheet[10] so I can turn her from side to side. I find that if I stand on top of the bed, I can pull Jane up the bed so she can still have a blurry view of the tree outside the window.

Over the weekend a succession of different community nurses visit to refill the syringe drivers. Jane waits peacefully. Her mother and younger sister want to visit again on the Sunday and although Jane has decreed no more visitors, we can hardly refuse. The scientific cousin wants to visit but cannot get to Edinburgh until Monday. Off stage her mother and I communicate about the realities she might face, but she is determined to come and Jane wants to see her. Drawing on evidence from her study of patients facing death, Copp (1998) proposes that the dying experience is an awareness of a separation between the body and the person (self). While acknowledging that her theory is largely hypothetical, she suggests that some may experience a sense of the body being ready for death when the person is not. I have a sense that Jane is waiting, hanging on, for the visit of her young cousin. There is a determination in her despite her clearly dying state. Yet, I have my doubts she will last, but I try to remain optimistic; that evening I email my sister:

> Here it's been another day on the downhill bobsleigh with HRH getting more happy mixture in her pump this morning and then being very drowsy all day. However, [the scientific cousin] came up for a visit which we didn't think she would manage in time but Jane was really pleased that she did. Yesterday [Jane's mother and younger sister] came through which wasn't easy but everyone was glad they did. It's particularly hard when people come to say goodbye although [the scientific cousin], who's just turned 21, was very adult, kind and strong. Anyway, when I've finished my wee dram, even though it's a school night, I'd better go to bed as you never know when you're going to need to spring into coherent action around here.
>
> *(Personal email, 21 May 2012)*

Now, as I write it is five years since Jane became ill and although my memories of Jane's final hours still seem clear they are not as vivid as they once were. I used the email quotation as a prompt in the storyboard to be asked about Jane's death in the last interview. However, the interviewer's interest centred on the last visits of Jane's family. We both became upset and the interview was paused. After I explained that I had not been able to describe the end which is a necessary conclusion to the story, we restarted:

INTERVIEWER: Can you say a bit about how that went, after [the scientific cousin] had visited.

VA: She left mid-afternoon and I continued to check [Jane] was okay and that she was comfortable. She was mostly just breathing heavily and drifting in and out of sleep. I didn't feel I needed to stay at her side, she knew I could see her from the living room and that I could hear the slightest thing. So I spent a quiet evening, lots of people kept sending texts, her sisters, close friends and I had various little reassuring messages to send that she was comfortable and it was okay.

Eventually I went to bed and I was up a couple of times during the night. Between three and four she was quite nauseated again and I was giving her hyoscine which was making her mouth dry. Each time when I got up, I turned her to the other side and so about four I'd got back into bed and fell asleep. I remember waking up very suddenly, shortly after seven, and looked at her and she was dead. I think I possibly woke up with her last breath. I didn't want to watch her die, to keep wondering if that was the last breath. I knew that I would wake with the slightest thing.

(Interview Eleven, 5 November 2013)

Finally, 343 days after the train journey when I first noticed that there might be something seriously wrong with Jane, she has died from advanced ovarian cancer. The final month was as she wanted, at home with me and our two cats. Family and friends were in close contact, visiting as she withdrew from public life. She directed the dance to the end, clear in her desires and wishes.

The Dance to Death, the narrative account of the Illness Period, has been presented with reference to relevant literature using a style that draws on that suggested by *embodied relational understanding* (Todres & Galvin, 2008). In the three chapters with their nine stories there are two turning points, the first in *Turning*[11] when Jane visits the herbalist and takes active responsibility for her situation. The second comes in *Reviewing*,[12] following the laparoscopy, when active treatment of her disease gives way to palliation. There is an apparent shift in the narrative as the medical voice from the health records fades away to be replaced by Jane's enthusiasm for the exquisite. The final chapter now revisits aspects of the Illness Period to consider the evidence for an aesthetic experience of dying and the return enhanced.

Notes

1. See for example the guidance for NHS England at www.nhs.uk/NHSEngland/thenhs/records/healthrecords/Pages/what_to_do.aspx and Health Rights Information Scotland at www.nhsinform.scot/care-support-and-rights/health-rights/access/health-records#accessing-your-health-records
2. http://ico.org.uk/for_the_public/topic_specific_guides/health
3. www.nhs.uk/NHSEngland/thenhs/records/healthrecords/Pages/overview.aspx
4. See www.macmillan.org.uk/Cancerinformation/Cancertypes/Ovary/Aboutovariancancer/Theovaries.aspx for an example of such a stylised diagram.
5. This a reference to the revolting scene in the Monty Python film, *The Meaning of Life*, when the morbidly obese and glutinous character Monsieur Creosote explodes (see Michael, 2013 for gory details).
6. The accumulation of fluid in the abdominal cavity as a result of neoplastic disease (Parsons et al., 1996).
7. Father of the composer Felix and a German philosopher and to whom the founding of the Jewish enlightenment is sometimes attributed (Arkush, 2007).
8. The normal range is 115–165 g/L.
9. This proved to be an urban myth and I am not sure where the idea originated. However, it was the chemotherapy that caused Jane's heightened olfactory awareness and altered sense of taste (Bernhardson et al., 2009).
10. I was unaware of such innovations as they did not exist in the 1980s.
11. See Chapter 3.
12. See Chapter 4.

References

Adamson, Veronica (2015) *The Dance to Death: The Aesthetic Experience of Dying*, PhD Thesis, Edinburgh: University of Edinburgh
Al-Ubaydli, Mohammed (2012) 'Patients must have control of their medical records', *British Medical Journal*, 345, e5575
Arkush, A (2007) 'The liberalism of Moses Mendelssohn' in M L Morgan & P E Gordon, Eds, *The Cambridge Companion to Modern Jewish Philosophy*, Cambridge: Cambridge University Press, 35–52
Bernhardson, Britt-Marie, Tishelman, Carol & Rutqvist, Lars Erik (2009) 'Olfactory changes among patients receiving chemotherapy', *European Journal of Oncology Nursing*, 13, 1, 9–15
Copp, Gina (1998) 'A review of current theories of death and dying', *Journal of Advanced Nursing*, 28, 2, 382–390
Davies, Peter (2012) 'Should patients be able to control their own records?', *British Medical Journal*, 345, e4905
Eng, Donna S & Lee, Joyce M (2013) 'The promise and peril of mobile health applications for diabetes and endocrinology', *Pediatric Diabetes*, 14, 231–238
Eskander, Ramez N & Tewari, Krishnansu S (2012) 'Emerging treatment options for management of malignant ascites in patients with ovarian cancer', *International Journal of Women's Health*, 4, 395–404
Fleming, N D, Alvarez-Secord, A, Von Gruenigen, V, Miller, M J & Abernethy, A P (2009) 'Indwelling catheters for the management of refractory malignant ascites: a systematic literature overview and retrospective chart review', *Journal of Pain Symptom Management*, 38, 3, 341–349
Frank, Arthur W (2001) 'Can we research suffering?', *Qualitative Health Research*, 11, 353–362
Friberg, F, Andersson, E P & Bengtsson, J (2007) 'Pedagogical encounters between nurses and patients in a medical ward – a field study', *International Journal of Nursing Studies*, 44, 534–544
Froggatt, Katherine (1997) 'Rites of passage and the hospice culture', *Mortality*, 2, 123–136
Froggatt, Katherine (1998) 'The place of metaphor and language in exploring nurses' emotional work', *Journal of Advanced Nursing*, 28, 2, 332–338
Furber, Lynn (2010) *Investigating Interactions: How do Doctors and Patients Experience the Disclosure of Significant Information in the Advanced Cancer Setting and How do these Experiences Enhance Practice?*, PhD thesis, Nottingham: University of Nottingham
Greenberg, J, Pyszczynski, T & Solomon, S (1986) 'The causes and consequences of a need for self-esteem: a Terror Management Theory', in R F Baumeister, Ed., *Public Self and Private Self*, New York: Springer-Verlag
Hatch, K D, Beecham, J D, Blessing, J A & Creasman, W T (1991) 'Responsiveness of patients with advanced ovarian carcinoma to tamoxifen', *Cancer*, 68, 2, 269–271
Hovey, Richard & Craig, Robert (2011) 'Understanding the relational aspects of learning with, from, and about the other', *Nursing Philosophy*, 12, 262–270
Innes, S & Payne, S (2009) 'Advanced cancer patients' prognostic information preferences: a review', *Palliative Medicine*, 23, 29–39
Kipps, E, Tan, D S & Kaye, S B (2013) 'Meeting the challenge of ascites in ovarian cancer: new avenues for therapy and research', *Nature Review Cancer*, 13, 4, 273–282
Kmietowicz, Zosia (2012) 'Cancer patients should have access to device to treat fluid retention at home, says NICE', *British Medical Journal*, 344, e2272
Macdonald, R, Kirwan, J, Roberts, S, Gray, D, Allsopp, L & Green, J (2006) 'Ovarian cancer and ascites: a questionnaire on current management in the United Kingdom', *Journal of Palliative Medicine*, 9, 6, 1264–1270
McCreaddie, Mary & Wiggins, Sally (2008) 'The purpose and function of humour in health, health care and nursing: a narrative review', *Journal of Advanced Nursing*, 61, 6, 584–595

Mercadante, S, Intravaia, G, Ferrera, P, Villari, P & David, F (2008) 'Peritoneal catheter for continuous drainage of ascites in advanced cancer patients', *Support Care Cancer*, 16, 8, 975–978

Michael, Chris (2013) 'How we made Monty Python's *The Meaning of Life*', *The Guardian*, Film, 30 September

Parsons, S L, Watson, S A & Steele, R J C (1996) 'Malignant ascites', *British Journal of Surgery*, 83, 1, 6–14

Rankin, Janet M & Campbell, Marie (2009) 'Institutional ethnography (IE), nursing work and hospital reform: IE's cautionary analysis', *Forum: Qualitative Social Research*, 10, 2

Rolfe, Gary (1998) 'The theory–practice gap in nursing: from research-based practice to practitioner-based research', *Journal of Advanced Nursing*, 28, 3, 672–679

Samuels, A, Shorter, B & Plaut, F (1986) *A Critical Dictionary of Jungian Analysis*, London: Routledge

Scottish Government, The (2012) *eHealth Strategy 2011–2017*, Edinburgh: The Scottish Government

Smith, D E (2005) *Institutional Ethnography: A Sociology for People*, Lanham: AltaMira Press

Smolle, E, Taucher, V & Haybaeck, J (2014) 'Malignant ascites in ovarian cancer and the role of targeted therapeutics', *Anticancer Research*, 34, 4, 1553–1561

Smyth, Dion (2011) 'Black humour in health care: a laughing matter?', *International Journal of Palliative Nursing*, 17, 11, 523

Smyth, J F, Gourley, C, Walker, G, MacKean, M J, Stevenson, A, Williams, A R, Nafussi, A A, Rye, T, Rye, R, Stewart, M, McCurdy, J, Mano, M, Reed, N, McMahon, T, Vasey, P, Gabra, H & Langdon, S P (2007) 'Antiestrogen therapy is active in selected ovarian cancer cases: the use of letrozole in estrogen receptor-positive patients', *Clinical Cancer Research*, 13, 12, 3617–3622

Stanojević, Z, Rančić, G, Radić, S, Potic-Zečević, N, Dordević, B, Marković, M & Todorovska, I (2004) 'Pathogenesis of malignant ascites in ovarian cancer patients', *Archive of Oncology*, 12, 2, 115–118

Starling, Ernest H (1896) 'On the absorption of fluids from the connective tissue spaces', *Journal of Physiology*, 19, 4, 312–326

Stephenson, J & Gilbert, J (2002) 'The development of clinical guidelines on paracentesis for ascites related to malignancy', *Palliative Medicine*, 16, 3, 213–218

Tapping, C R, Ling, L & Razack, A (2012) 'PleurX drain use in the management of malignant ascites: safety, complications, long-term patency and factors predictive of success', *British Journal of Radiology*, 85, 1013, 623–628

Taylor, Shelley E (1983) 'Adjustment to threatening events: a theory of cognitive adaptation', *American Psychologist*, 38, 1161–1173

The, Anne-Mei (2002) *Palliative Care and Communication: Experiences in the Clinic*, Milton Keynes: Open University Press

Todres, Les & Galvin, Kathleen T (2008) 'Embodied interpretation: a novel way of evocatively re-presenting meanings in phenomenological research', *Qualitative Research*, 8, 5, 568–583

Turner, Victor (1969) *The Ritual Process*, Ithaca: Cornell University Press

Watson, Katie (2011) 'Gallows humor in medicine', *Hastings Center Report*, 41, 5, 37–45

Weinman, J, Yusuf, G, Berks, R, Rayner, S & Petrie, K J (2009) 'How accurate is patients' anatomical knowledge: a cross-sectional, questionnaire study of six patient groups and a general public sample', *BMC Family Practice*, 10

WHO, World Health Organization (1990) *Cancer Pain Relief and Palliative Care*, Geneva: World Health Organization

WHO, World Health Organization (2004) *Palliative Care: Symptom Management and End-of-life Care*, Geneva: World Health Organization

5
THE AESTHETIC EXPERIENCE OF DYING

This book has centred on three themes: a life limited by illness, aesthetic experience and the return enhanced. The concept of the return enhanced has also been prominent in the natural cycle of research and the writing process. Initially it was unclear how this particular interpretation of German philosophy could work in this study. In this final chapter, the dynamic process of binary synthesis as one of tension, intensity and resolution is set in a wider context. The tension of Jane's dying has been resolved as the rhythmic patterns of the lifeworld have been understood through the process of reflecting on the experience.

A contemplative narrative of suffering

To understand what happened to Jane and to us as life partners, it seemed necessary to tell many stories from the Illness Period. The extracts used range from minimalist, one word headings to more explicit accounts of particular events and episodes. In an early draft of the thesis I wrote that I wanted the reader to have a strong sense of the visceral reality of advanced cancer and its poisonous treatment. However, in comparison with others who have written of their personal experience, particularly of ovarian cancer (Rose, 1995; Gubar, 2012), this version seems quite mild. My audience is primarily the academic community; Jane's blog post readers were her fans: the social network of family, friends and former colleagues solicitous for news of her progress. Our dissimilar purposes require different styles. Mine attempts an embodied interpretation of a shared experience which is in parts uncomfortable. Jane's style is witty, humorous with dashes of dark truths edged with light relief. In constructing and analysing the narrative account I had wanted to create a "pedagogy of suffering" (Frank, 2013: 145) as something from which society could learn. Yet she rarely wrote about her illness and suffering, instead her narrative is like Frank's account of Miss Tod as "simply being" (Frank, 2013: 211).

What finally emerges is a more contemplative account. In this final chapter I re-explore some of the stories from *The Dance to Death* and compare them first with reference to Frank's typology of illness narratives (Frank, 2013) and then in contrast with other similar illness writings.

In the study corpus only five of Jane's thirty-four blog posts are specifically about her illness. There are references to it in others but as an aside and not as the focus. The story she really tells in the Illness Period is not one of suffering and disruption but of a life well lived. However, before I elaborate on this point, I want to outline my conceptualisation of suffering. Previously I believed suffering was an indication of failure on the part of carers, whether professional or lay. If a sick person was suffering then in a simplistic sense, someone had not cared for them correctly. Insufficient pain relief had been given or pillows had not been properly plumped: the doctrine of my nurse training. Conventionally, suffering is understood in terms of pain and its negation, and to be unwell. Yet the medical model can be impotent to suffering that is not directly connected to a particular illness or disease (Frank, 2001). In this indefinable sense "To suffer is to lose your grip. Suffering is expressed in myth as the wound that does not kill but cannot be healed" (Frank, 2001: 355). This suggests a sense of permanence as a scar from an experience that has been endured and a pedagogical interpretation of suffering as "what the ill have to teach society" (Frank, 2013: 145). It was in this sense that I first explored the narrative accounts of Jane's illness as she endured it and as I had witnessed it. However, a more contemplative approach goes beyond clinical reasoning to look at the moral aspects of events for their inherent goodness (Mattingly, 1998a), to appreciate the process of the return enhanced. By returning to the difficult experience of Jane's illness and her dying, my understanding has been enhanced by dwelling in that place with the coherent integration and not active separation (Galvin & Todres, 2007) of clinical reasoning with the practice of the 'best good' (Mattingly, 1998a: 291). Now I conceptualise suffering as both existential and physical, knowing both can be addressed through care and compassion. During Jane's final weeks she did suffer physically but she managed her existential pain by sitting on her rock waiting to walk through the waterfall beyond.

Narrating illness

If life can be well lived despite suffering ill health, "how will I find ways to avoid feeling that my life is diminished by illness and eventually dying?" (Frank, 2013: xvi). The term 'bucket list', popularised primarily through the 2007 film[1] of the same name, has become the "companion story" (Frank, 2010: 43) to guide those facing a diagnosis of life-limiting illness. This is the wish list of life experiences deemed most essential before premature death and foregrounds the quest for life to be undiminished by illness. Frank derived his concept of companion stories from two ideas. Firstly, stories are performative materials (Law, 2000) capable of shape-shifting in their re-telling. The second aspect, that they are inherently evolutionary, was inspired by Donna Haraway's manifesto on companion species. She argues that dogs are a typical companion species which has evolved from the wolf into the domestic friend to whom many are now "bonded in significant otherness" (Haraway, 2003: 16). The two essential features of companion stories are firstly that similar stories shape one another in a process of coevolution. Secondly, companion stories take care of each other through this shaping process (Frank, 2010). The phrase 'bucket list' is a derivation of the slang expression 'to kick the bucket'. However, the bucket in this sense has its origins in the old French word for balance, meaning a yoke or beam, on which anything could be hung (*SOED*, 2007). Neither of these expressions are stories as such, but they are signifiers of stories about death and dying. Telling a story about kicking the bucket could be an irreverent way of disclosing the death of an acquaintance. A bucket list story might tell of a young person who manages to pack many exciting experiences into a life foreshortened by cancer. As a type of story it would belong to the genre of epic, as 'things to see/do/witness/taste before you die'.

For us, a bucket list is never mentioned, instead Jane notes "Last Thursday we achieved another tick on our 'Things to do in Edinburgh' list with a visit to the zoo" (Blog post, 'A Day at the Zoo', day 137). The list is not discussed but exists in Jane's head. She has a particular preference for ordering tasks as a checklist which is then awarded ticks in a manner reminiscent of a sticky star from a school teacher. In another blog post she lists various cultural events we have attended. Life is being lived at full tilt:

> There's no doubting our social life is much improved since we've been living in Edinburgh. This has more to do with how isolated we had become in our Highland village, than with a full diary of glittering events. But by our standards we've been pretty busy. We've ticked quite a lot off our 'things to do in Edinburgh' list.
>
> *(Blog post, 'Social Life', day 187)*

The blog post goes on to list cultural highlights, visits to monuments, art galleries and outings in general. Before we met, Jane had been an enthusiastic hill walker, having scaled more than half of the Scottish Munros. As a keen, though less gallous walker, I had previously found the perfect hills in the Pentlands, to the south of Edinburgh. My first real hill walks were there with my mother. We revelled in the delight of being so near to the city while in the middle of a grouse moor. Jane is honest with her initial view, "Purists may mock the Pentlands (I used to) and draw invidious comparisons with classic west coast ridge walks" (Blog post, 'Small hills and sock mountains', day 106). One of the attractions of the flat is "Our living room has grand views of Capelaw and Allermuir Hills in the Pentlands (which are definitely to be ascended ere long)" (Blog post, 'Indoor Camping', day 62). This is a life not so much diminished by illness as one that has accommodated it.

Being in, with or near nature is a recurrent theme in many blog entries. Even while recovering from the initial diagnostic laparoscopy, Jane wants more than just fresh air:

It took a few days to recover so that was just small walks maybe just round the block. Then I took her in the car to the nearby park and walking round the pond. She drew such strength from being out in the fresh air, from seeing birds. She wanted to see nature, to see birds, to see plants, to see trees and to be out in the countryside.

(Interview Two, 13 August 2013)

In Edinburgh, visits to the Botanic Gardens are a regular feature to assuage clinic visits or the enforced inactivity of a treatment session "The day before the first [chemo] session [Veronica] took me to commune with the yew trees" (Blog post, 'Silver Linings', day 45). The symbolism of yew trees as the source of the chemotherapy agent, Taxol, was noted earlier. We both use the gardens as a living reference for plants and trees, sharing a common interest in horticulture. In turn this aesthetic pleasure is shared with others:

We took [my brother and partner] to the Botanic Gardens and showed them all our favourite trees. There's something particularly special about showing a special place to someone else and appreciating their appreciation.

(Blog post, 'Portobello', day 47)

When she starts to feel the treatment is having a beneficial effect, the walks become braver:

This morning we climbed to the top of Allermuir Hill, the focal point of our living room view. Only 1619 feet high but all achievements are relative and I was very pleased to make it to the top and back down again, feeling stronger and more like myself with every step. The wind was exhilarating to the point of almost blowing us off our feet and the southern Pentland ridge emerging tantalising as we climbed promises much exciting walking to come.

(Blog post, 'Top of the View', day 89)

Two months on and into the now weekly chemo regime, her enthusiasm remains undiminished:

We had another grand walk in the Pentlands last weekend – 12 km through the Green Cleugh to Scald Law. Sunshine, blue sky and light winds, slight autumn nip in the air, crisp burnished colour all around. It felt really good to be on a genuine expedition, returning to the car as the sun was disappearing into the west and the sky was turning from pale blue to indigo.

(Blog post, 'Bimbling Along', day 150)

The connection to and participation in nature is paramount; illness is transcended, diminished and almost forgotten by the exhilaration of climbing a hill. Jane views a bigger, wider world with distant vistas and far horizons; her insignificance and situation can be seen in context. This is Jane's real bucket, the beam on which she balances life with death. Her accounts of nature and the landscape are not confined to the macro world of hills and valleys but imbued with details of birds spotted, flowers sniffed and trees beheld. These are her companion stories of living life, reinforced in the pleasure of telling the story. Yet if she is a storyteller wounded (Frank, 2013) by disease, are her stories really just a simple nature notebook to assuage the severity of her illness? These accounts also exemplify a *return enhanced*. The interplay between the intense appreciation of the effulgent experience of nature in counterpoint to the darkness of disease.

Conventionally, the call for stories in response to illness may serve two purposes: as reparation for the damage of the illness to the self, and secondly as a repository for the public news broadcasting system (Frank, 2013). Previously I believed Jane's use was the latter, her mechanism for keeping the support circle apprised. However perhaps the more essential purpose was a self-maintaining function. Story-making is a craft act of shaping and honing that can entertain and distract an active mind for hours. It was what enabled her to sit passively through long treatment sessions or hours of recuperation on her couch throne. From either a view was essential "I sat in a reclining chair by an open window above a flower garden" (Blog post, 'Silver Linings', day 45) and "certainly a huge relief to be writing this from my throne by the window with my view of the hills" (Blog post, 'Breaking out of the Hospice', day 323). In the first quotation she is enduring treatment and in the second enjoying the sanctity of literal *at-homeness* (Galvin & Todres, 2011b). On both occasions, story-making was her companion. Later in this chapter I will investigate the work that stories do. Here it is worth noting that while storytelling is a dual act of reaffirmation (Frank, 2013) for both the self and others, there is a prior stage as "Jane was very good at rehearsing what she wanted to say" (Interview Two, 13 August 2013). It is not possible to access the inner workings of embryonic stories but the process of story-making may be at least as important as the product.

Working stories

Frank's influential work on narratives of illness (Woods, 2012) has come to define how such accounts are now interpreted and understood. He identifies three story types, restitution, chaos and quest, all of which can be told in an illness:

> Restitution stories attempt to outdistance mortality by rendering illness transitory. Chaos stories are sucked into the undertow of illness and the disasters that attend it. Quest stories meet suffering head on; they accept illness and seek to use it.
>
> *(Frank, 2013: 115)*

Once the typology is known, it becomes difficult not to then view illness stories through these lenses and they interpellate as we are "made to constitute our objects in particular ways" (Law, 2000: 16). However, before expanding on this typology, other interpretations merit consideration. Robinson (1990) sought to address the ambivalence with which personal illness accounts were viewed at that time despite the quality of the deeply meaningful content and the insight provided into the experience of illness. He notes "these very qualities seem to make any systematic, valid and reliable attempts to create generalisable propositions difficult, if not impossible" (Robinson, 1990: 1173).

In contrast, the relational aspects of the narrator, the narrative and the illness are recognised by Hydén (1997) who emphasises that the three may not necessarily be one and the same. An account of the personal experience of illness will combine all three to produce a story of illness as narrative. So a medical account will convey a narrative about the illness between professionals. In the account here the relational aspects are evident in *The Dance to Death* where Jane and I narrate her illness *as* a narrative interspersed with additional accounts *about* her illness narrated by various health professionals. My purpose here is not a sociological interpretation of chronic illness as related through researcher interviews. It is to understand the autobiographical nature of life during an illness experience and the relationship between the different stories told about that experience. Frank's typology provides a useful framework for the interpretation of self-generated, as opposed to research-occasioned, accounts of living with and beside an illness experience.

Narrative accounts, as a set of stories not only intersect but also interfere with each other (Law, 2000). Connections may be found in similar stories but there may be a disorderly aspect such as when a temporal sequence is either misremembered or perhaps has its chronology deliberately distorted for some other reason. However, it can be difficult for the intended audience to follow a story if its telling is too disordered, so some organisation into, for example foreground and background, is necessary. Frank (2010) suggests there is some fine-tuning to do to the work stories which involves the use of a default guidance system with two axes. The first axis connects personal understanding with affiliations, while the second connects what can be good about life with what makes it dangerous (Frank, 2010: 48). The following extract illustrates the system in action:

> the oncologist broke the news ... that the CT scan showed the tumour had not apparently shrunk very much ... He asked if this news surprised me. I think I nodded, while actually it would be more accurate to say that it rather floored me. Because I had been feeling so much better, and stronger, I was sure the chemo was working and that surgery would be scheduled soon.
>
> *(Blog post, 'A Different Mindset', day 98)*

The first personal-affiliation axis receives the news of the CT scan results by using a coping story of appearing to be in unsurprised agreement (nodding) while concealing the real response. The second good-dangerous axis reveals the misleading nature of feeling better and raising expectations while hiding reality. The full version of this quotation appears in the story *Treating*[2] where the interpretation focused on the sequence of events and their effect on Jane. The analysis there was on the *content* of the story, not on the *work* of the story.

Frank's restitution story is founded on the statement "Yesterday I was healthy, today I'm sick, tomorrow I'll be healthy again" (Frank, 2013: 77). It serves to distance mortality and reinforce belief in the efficacy of the medical treatment. The chaos story is in sharp contrast to and opposite from restitution. It is hard to hear an experience without sequence or causality that "traces the edges of a wound that can only be told around" (Frank, 2013: 98). Reading tales of restitution and chaos can be difficult, hard work for the reader. Quest stories are more comfortable as they offer a coherent account of acceptance and distancing the chaotic disruption of illness. They utilise illness as "the occasion of a journey that becomes a quest" (Frank, 2013: 115), or the Bildung[3] of the Bildungsroman. Quest stories are the type with the greatest range in the genre of illness stories. Frank elaborates on this aspect in two ways. First, as the narrative structure of a heroic journey with its three stages of departure, initiation and return "best described by Joseph Campbell in his classic work, *The Hero with a Thousand Faces*" (Frank, 2013: 117). The second way in which Frank extends the specification of quest stories is by suggesting they may have three different facets: memoir, manifesto and automythology (Frank, 2013: 119).

The memoir is perhaps the easiest form in its depiction of life with the incorporation of illness. Pathography is a term used to describe a published account of the hopes and fears of living with illness (Hawkins, 1999). Such books may also act as a guide to treatment and help to shape the reader's understanding of the course of the disease. In a review of her earlier book, *Reconstructing Illness: Studies in Pathography* (Hawkins, 1993), Frank (2013) notes that the most popular pathographies have celebrity authors, which raises issues of voyeurism and the commodification of the illness experience, that is to benefit financially from the story. Nevertheless, Frank finds illness memoirs to be the most gentle of the quest narratives as their popularity with the public appears to confirm.

The manifesto type of quest story is the opposite of the memoir and therefore generally makes uncomfortable reading. The style is usually emancipatory, giving a voice to suffering and the truth of illness that must be told. Susan Gubar's *Memoir of a Debulked Woman: Enduring Ovarian Cancer* (Gubar, 2012) is part memoir and part manifesto in its telling of one academic's account of her personal suffering and surgical evisceration. I found it too uncomfortable to read and too close for comfort. I have read excerpts, feeling galled and frustrated by her brutal honesty. While I can empathise with her plight and respect her sincerity, I am uncertain who the intended audience would be for such a work. It is a testament of survival and raises the issue of public awareness of the disease, but I would not recommend it to a woman with ovarian cancer. However, reading some of the online reviews of the book suggests that sufferers, carers and many others, do find the text inspiring and helpful. Thompson (2007) suggests that women with ovarian cancer want to talk with fellow sufferers and will therefore seek women whom they feel are able "to hear as well as provide recognition" (Thompson, 2007: 347). The third type of quest is the automythological type and tells a story of reinvention as an illness response. It is more than mere survival, it is rebirth. It can be recognised by the use of powerful language, such as destiny and regeneration, to tell legends and mythological interpretations of the illness course.

Frank's (2013) real purpose in proposing his typology is not to suggest a general unifying type but to assist the reader in 'listening' to the story. I have admitted my own difficulty in reading illness stories so how does the typology help to listen to Jane's story? Before I address this question, there is another point to note "In any illness, *all* three narrative types are told, alternatively and repeatedly" (Frank, 2013: 76, original emphasis). Similarly, Bury asserts "whatever narrative form may be identified in analysis, many accounts move from one to another" (Bury, 2001: 280). In my overwhelming desire to tell the story of Jane's illness, I did not attempt to analyse Jane's blog posts. This is not an excuse but a feature of the emergent nature of the study as a contemplative inquiry. However, Frank makes a valid point and examples of all three narrative types can be heard in Jane's writing.

Listening to Jane's stories

The blog post 'Silver Linings' (day 45) was the longest and written three weeks after diagnosis. The opening paragraph[4] accords with the literal definition of the restitution story. This is exemplified in the three phrase sentence which begins *Yesterday I was healthy*, and Jane writes: "Our little world turned upside down and it's taken a wee while before I've felt able to write about what's been happening." It is the first clause, the world of health turned upside down to ill health that signifies the start of restitution. The second phrase, *today I'm sick*, follows immediately in her next sentence "In short: I've been diagnosed with ovarian cancer", and is self-explanatory. The final phrase, *tomorrow I'll be healthy again*, comes after a blog page of diagnostic tests and procedures. "Treatment is to be four cycles of chemotherapy in the first instance, which they hope will shrink the tumour to an operable size, then a hysterectomy." In telling this restitution story, Jane is distancing herself from her own mortality, despite her explicit description of the extent of the disease "I have a Stage 3 serous tumour which started on my left ovary, has munched its way through most of my uterus and 'involves' the bladder wall and the rectum". Her focus is on being restored to health by the treatment plan.

However, there are also traces of the edge of chaos, the second illness narrative plot type, suggested by the delay in writing the account of what has happened. Following the uncomfortable business trip to London, she writes "After a couple of sleepless nights we decided something had to be done." Her reader is spared my recollection "She was miserable with the pain in her back, with the tightness in her abdomen, with the feeling unwell" (Interview One, 9 July 2013) and diary entry "Woke me at 4.30am in severe pain" (Personal diary, day 3). Jane was too conscious of her audience and the informative intention of the blog to write anything that might cause additional anxiety and upset. At the time I had a strong sense that '*no one*' (Frank, 2013: 101, original emphasis) was in control. We felt out of control not knowing what was wrong with Jane; when help was sought, respite was temporary. Jane's account ignores the chaos by adhering to narrative format as sequence and consequence (Riessman & Speedy, 2007), diverting attention to the 'lovely young doctors'. Chaos is the embodiment of suffering and can only be described by the sufferer in oblique terms. It was perhaps because the chaotic aspects were not told by Jane that I felt that there was something missing from her narrative that needed to be told, that I had to tell.

In effect, part of my role as her primary carer was at best to prevent anything chaotic occurring, but if it seemed imminent then to absorb and deal with it. A difficulty may then arise for the carer when they do not have time to resolve their experience of chaos. It becomes their embodiment of their partner's disease. There are two other explanations for the lack of chaos in Jane's account: first she was all too aware of the sensibilities of her audience. And second, as Riessman has recently observed through her own personal experience, "Omissions are one way to exercise control over the uncontrollable" (Riessman, 2015: 8). So when the chaotic does happen, Jane does not write of the experience herself. One particularly chaotic episode was the insertion of the permanent abdominal drain, described in *Reviewing*.[5] Chaos ensued when the attendant staff chose not to heed my advice that Jane should not be laid completely flat. They did, she vomited, everyone flapped. If the chaos story is "an anti-narrative, so it is a non-self story" (Frank, 2013: 105), it is then neutralised when a coherent story is told. In Jane's version of the drain insertion, there is no suggestion of chaos nor of her suffering during the procedure. Instead she writes "I now have a permanent drain fitted which makes 'little and often' drainage possible" (Blog post, 'Catching Up', day 272). This could be read as a restitution story but Jane's interpretation is more likely to have been as a binary synthesis of chaos being subordinated by order.

The third illness narrative type, the quest story, is the most complicated as the illness is expressed as a journey with different facets to its plot structure. There may be memoir with the inclusion of life outwith the illness, or manifesto which strives to reveal the truth of the illness, while automythology occasions the reinvention of the ill self (Frank, 2013). Quest narratives enable the sick person to tell their story. In a restitution narrative the action is with the treatment regime; in a chaos story the self is consumed by the suffering and cannot tell, but with a quest the story is in the foreground. Consequently they are the most common type of published illness accounts using a narrative structure to provide a framework for the sick person to accept their illness and find an alternative way of being. The predominant style in Jane's writing is that of memoir where she writes extensively about everyday life with occasional illness bulletins. She describes a figurative journey as a passage through a life that foregrounds the present but makes few references to the future. Perhaps this is because she soon realised there was little chance of remission or sustained restitution. Jane was teleported to Susan Sontag's "kingdom of the ill" (Sontag, 1978: 3); the expression is ironic in itself for someone who disliked illness metaphors. Once in this new place, it was interesting "Chemotherapy is a fascinating process" (Blog post, 'Silver Linings', day 45) but also engendered feelings of being "a bit tired and paranoid if anyone sneezes in my proximity" (Blog post,

'Silver Linings', day 45). This was not so much a land to journey through, as a place of work. Jane's new job was to balance the exhausting clinical interventions by sitting on her 'rock'. The work done in this place was healing self-restoration, making herself whole to assuage the effects of the illness and its treatment.

There are many examples in her blog of real journeys, the distance that can be travelled in a day, an outing or a day trip. Unsurprisingly, given her fondness for rugged landscapes and hill-walking, her preferred metaphor was "There are many ways up the mountain. Other people can help – describe the landscape, suggest routes, provide kit and provisions, accompany me for part of the way – but I take the path myself." (Blog post, 'A Different Mindset', day 89). This is where the temporal and situational context is helpful. This quotation comes early in the Illness Period when Jane was no longer relying on others to do the healing work. But she had to find a way to convey this change in direction to her readers. At the start of her illness Jane had devolved control to the health professionals. It took time for her to work through her internal, personal chaos before she could resume full control.

If the quest narrative is conceived as a heroic journey (Campbell, 1949/2012), the three stages of departure, initiation and return, equate with van Gennep's (1960) 'rites of passage' not least because Campbell made extensive use of the concept in his own work. Frank suggests a recursive process where "the journey is taken in order to find out what sort of journey one has been taking" (Frank, 2013: 117). In other words it is a quest to find purpose despite being ill. This suggests a reflective element, a story that is written at some later point perhaps after treatment, recovery or remission. My point is that Jane may have seen her collection of blog posts as a traveller's account of her journey through the time she was ill. However, while "illness narratives are by nature ambiguous because they do not have a clear and foreseeable end" (Hydén, 1997: 60), the ambiguity in Jane's story was magnified because it would end with her death. For Jane the blog was a bulletin board of her restoration work.

Manifesto stories are those that tell a prophetic truth. Frank (2013) uses Audre Lorde's account (Lorde, 1980) of her refusal to wear a prosthesis following a mastectomy as an example. In similar vein, Jane declined to wear a wig following her chemotherapy-induced alopecia:

> I'm now magnificently bald, by the way, although some grey fuzz has started to reappear which looks and feels a bit odd. A bit self-conscious, I've been alert to people's reactions – some give me a big broad smile, some look away, most don't seem to notice. Being bald is only a stigma for women, of course.
>
> *(Blog post, 'Indoor Camping', day 62)*

Jane's prophetic truth was to reaffirm herself as a woman and not as a cancer victim. Furthermore, the quest manifesto "asserts that illness is a social issue, not simply a personal affliction" (Frank, 2013: 122). Another way in which a quest manifesto can be interpreted is as a public policy statement as suggested by this:

One of the things we found most disconcerting about my cancer diagnosis was the official advice effectively banning vitamin supplements. We had what we then considered a pretty healthy and well-balanced diet, supplemented with a carefully researched and tailored regime of vitamins and minerals. It seemed counter-intuitive for me to stop all supplements immediately, at a time when my body was particularly vulnerable, on the basis that the medical profession had no evidence of the extent to which vitamins might interfere with the effects of the chemotherapy on the tumour. Spot the double negative? 'We don't know if it might not work'. When you're that scared rabbit in the headlights of the doctors and nurses and they are saying that vitamin C might encourage cancer cells to grow, and live yoghurt might introduce infection to your immunocompromised gut, you do what they tell you. More or less. At least to start with.

(Blog post, 'Coping with Chemo', day 159)

In this example, Jane has reclaimed her right to participate in her treatment in her own way. This is a call for a partnership approach to her care where she would be an active participant and not just a passive recipient of the treatment regime. It can be difficult to read illness stories as anything other than a sad tale of triumph over adversity or as a heroic battle. While the above excerpt is about fighting the good fight, it is also one of preservation. Saving and salvaging what remains of the disease and treatment ravaged body is a quest for living.

The final type of quest story is that of automythology where the storyteller does not simply survive their illness but is reborn in the process (Frank, 2013). There are two instances of reinvention in Jane's illness narrative. The first concerns her own creation, the chemo 'bunnet', a soft skull cap. It had a dual purpose: to keep her bald head warm and to provide some style for her otherwise bland appearance. In addition to the loss of head hair, chemotherapy-induced alopecia renders the entire body to a hairless state (Jayde et al., 2013). While this is hardly an issue for a clothed adult, the loss of eyebrows and eyelashes can be too stark a contrast, rendering the face featureless. By wearing a colourful little hat, Jane reinvented her appearance to reflect the colourful and amusing character that she was trying to maintain. The myth in this reinvention was that in reality, she found the lack of definition to her face unbearable if she saw her reflection in a mirror, bunnet or not.

The second example of myth-making had emerged quite naturally before she was ill "[Veronica] made Epiphany Cake on the appointed day, and it came to pass that I once again received the bean, so normal royal service has been resumed for the year to come" (Blog post, 'Festive Family Favourites', day 212). The cake is a European tradition that we had acquired in Belgium when Jane had received the bean the previous year. A cake containing a bean or small ceramic figure is made to celebrate the Christian festival of Epiphany. When the cake is cut, whoever receives the bean is king or queen for the following year. Belgian bakeries selling the cakes supply a gold paper crown for the royal personage. So, it was a family joke that became a useful metaphor for treating Jane in a special way. If she was queen, she had royal prerogative to command whatever she wished and to be attended by her loyal subjects. It was a myth that she willingly participated in and to some extent encouraged but never exploited. There are various references to Jane as queen or royalty in correspondence with my sister. Being royal had various advantages such as not being required to do household chores and always having first choice of outings or entertainment. In the later stages of the disease, when eating became difficult as a result of abdominal swelling, being royal made food whims and fancies easier.

> Sometimes my requests are reasonably adult (I want sushi), others amusingly childish (chips, cola, chocolate ice cream). I can spend much of the afternoon deciding whether I'd rather have my hot smoked salmon peppered or honeyed, and basil or chives in my avocado salsa (with chips of course).
> *(Blog post, 'Catching Up', day 291)*

All of these requests were indulged and provided a useful distraction from the grim reality of only being able to eat very small amounts. Interpretation of the myth also provides an insight into our respective roles as queen and heroic carer. I could cope with all that I had to do in caring for Jane if she was my queen and I was her loyal servant. We were "a relationship in which each understands herself as requiring completion by the other" (Frank, 2013: 150). I did not have to think of having empathy for Jane and her situation, we were interdependent in our mutual need for each other.

By using Frank's typology of illness narratives, other aspects of the stories recounted have been identified. However, some question the effect of using such a typology as it promotes a particular model of the self (Woods, 2011). Additionally, there is a normative assumption pervading the medical humanities that the drive for narrative is healthy and desirable. As a testimonial form, the creation and performance of the illness narrative allows the ill person to become "the hero of her own story" (Woods, 2011: 75). But what if narrative is mistaken for life (Woods, 2012) and silence is equally important? The core of Frank's typology suggests that restitution stories are used by those in denial and obligated to medicine. Illness is transformative when it is either as a quest for the better or the chaos of becoming worse (Woods, 2012). Yet not everyone facing illness is called to narrative and some argue it may not even be in our best interests (Strawson, 2004). To then misinterpret silence as narrative failure may be to miss the real phenomenological opportunity to understand illness through other forms of self-expression (Carel, 2011; Woods, 2011). Therefore, while Frank's typology has been useful here in 'listening' to other aspects of Jane's illness, its use was not "intended as a pigeon-holing device" (Mishler, 1995: 117) and was to learn instead from other approaches. I have suggested that Jane's narrative was one of restoration, as a counter-balance to her illness and its treatment. To read it wholly in Frank's terms would be to misinterpret it first as a restitution denial of illness and dying, then as a quest for living. But this would be to fall into the Buddhist attachment trap and be deluded by the illusory nature of her writing. She was in no doubt that she was dying and writing about living was not the illusion. However, some family members did interpret it as such and were then apparently shocked to learn of her imminent demise.

Illness stories in two voices

Jane and I knew we were fortunate to have each other but we were conscious that, for many people, facing a life foreshortened by illness was not so easy. Whether it be for family pressures, responsibilities as carers of children, ageing parents or some other reason, one half of a couple devoting themselves to the care of the other may be a luxury. Being *at home* was discussed earlier as central to the well-being of the sick person. Historically, the sick person was cared for at home, on occasion even surgical operations were performed in the bedroom. Health care became organised and institutional, not least to halt the spread of infectious diseases such as tuberculosis. Now the sick, frail or dying person is often cared for in an institutional context, sometimes in hospital but often a care home or hospice. The knowledge and confidence to provide nursing care in the home is a lost art. The solution to health care problems, both actual and anticipated, is increasingly pharmaceutical. The move towards consumerism in health care coupled with developments such as expert patient programmes are consistent with and not contrary to the interests of the pharmaceutical industry (Williams et al., 2011). Nowadays if you feel you have flu, you self medicate and continue working or possibly take a few days off work. But you are unlikely to be nursed at home until you feel well again.

At the end of life for those with solid metastatic tumours, there is evidence that chemotherapy treatment may continue to be offered and used despite the likelihood of a reduced quality and duration to life (Davis, 2015). The situation is compounded by public expectations of the efficacy of the latest treatments and the reality of what can be delivered by health care services. The demand for new anticancer drugs, despite their marginal benefits, can consume the limited research resources for other debilitating conditions. The focus on the pharmaceutical treatment of cancer has also meant that there is less research into other non-drug therapies (Davis, 2015). There are many ways in which the dying experience might be enhanced, both pharmaceutically and by other means. But enhancement is a contested term used "to denote going beyond treatment or health" (Williams et al., 2011: 718), to be better than just well, whatever that might mean. In this context the enhancement of death and dying may appear to be at odds with the therapeutic desires of the ill person and their family. However, the opportunities for a more aesthetic experience when near the end of life do exist but they are poorly understood and under researched.

In my explorations of narrative accounts of illness, I have been struck by the apparent lack of studies of collaborative writing in illness narratives. I am not referring to collaborations between researchers but those between the sick person and, ideally their partner, or primary carer. There do not appear to be any reported analyses of naturally occurring co-authored narrative accounts of illness. Studies have investigated the service user experience of palliative care provision (Cotterell, 2006; Cotterell et al., 2009) or the needs of the family carer in a palliative setting (Newbury, 2009; Payne et al., 2012). It has been suggested that emotionally charged narrative accounts of death and dying should be treated with caution during analysis as it is easy to drift from the emotional surface to drawing theoretical conclusions based on the emotional response of the investigator (Eva & Paley, 2006). Nevertheless, there is an increasing interest in joint interviewing (Morris, 2001; Polak & Green, 2015) and in the co-construction of illness narratives (Radcliffe et al., 2013). The presentation by the couple of a united front (Gerhardt, 1991) in response to the adversity of illness is a common feature although women tend to dominate discussions (Radcliffe et al., 2013).

In addition to the benefits of joint interviewing that includes the possibility of making sense of shared experience together (Mattingly, 1998b), the contextual nature of care practices are focused through the "foregrounding of the intersubjective and heteroglossic nature of illness experiences" (Sakellariou et al., 2013: 1567). Essentially, intersubjectivity is the shared experience of lifeworlds which can extend into the adoption of others' language or heteroglossia. For example, in the blog post 'Silver Linings' when Jane first describes her illness, she uses clinical and anatomical language, and by the end the intersubjective nature of our relationship has been detailed and then summarised as "We're a team, and we are a winning team" (Blog post, 'Silver Linings', day 45). While similarities can be identified from joint interview studies, I was looking for consciously co-authored accounts that were more in the style of collective biography (Davies & Gannon, 2012). This form of collaborative writing and biographical memory work has developed over the past decade. As a method, it "does not look for a uni-directional oppressive effect of *discourse* on *individuals*. Rather, [it] is conceived as emergent in each moment, moments that are simultaneously discursive, relational, and material" (Davies & Gannon, 2012: 359, original emphasis).

To date, no studies have been identified of co-created accounts of patient and partner/carer narratives. Instead, I have drawn on two published examples of collective writing to illustrate the potential of such processes. The first is a co-authored book, *Cancer in Two Voices* by Sandra Butler and Barbara Rosenblum (1991). It tells the story of the personal relationship between two women; the focus is on Barbara's breast cancer diagnosis, treatment and death. The book was created by Sandra (Sandy) from their journals, diaries and letters, after Barbara's death. The second example was published as two separate books and as newspaper articles in *The Observer*.[6] The art critic Tom Lubbock's *Until Further Notice, I Am Alive* (2012) is his personal account of life with glioma, a brain tumour, and its effects on his language. His wife, the artist Marion Coutts, describes the eighteen months leading up to his death in *The Iceberg: A Memoir* (2014). She also wrote the introduction to Tom's book (Lubbock, 2012) and played a vital role in assisting him in his desire to write "about my life in public form" (Lubbock, 2012: 135).

The extracts are of necessity brief but they convey the essential nature of the co-created illness narrative. Both Barbara and Tom were aware of the advanced stage of their diseases at diagnosis. I have selected excerpts that illustrate the turning point when they each turn full face to death and also as reflected in their partner's accounts. Sandy and Barbara had decided to go on one last holiday to Florence but the exertion was hard for Barbara as Sandy recalls:

> The next day Barbara collapsed from exhaustion. We had left our hotel at dawn to watch the city awaken. Before long I realised that, inadvertently, we had gone too far … Barbara barely managed to stumble back to the hotel, needing to rest at every corner. She slept most of the remainder of the day, awakening near midnight. As we lay in each other's arms, she talked about her fear and her sense of missed opportunities … When we both awoke the next morning, fresh from our dreams, we understood we had moved imperceptibly closer to the inevitability of this ending, her death.
> (Butler & Rosenblum, 1991: 123)

A few days later Barbara writes:

> There has been a change in my medical status. Cancer is growing again in my liver. The symptoms are pretty terrible. I have more fatigue than ever before. A profound loss of energy and direction and an inability to be 'present'. I'm more detached, perhaps saying my good-byes in a way. I am just doing what is necessary to survive. My mind and body are doing what they – I – need to do. I cannot stay with my feelings so much. My awareness clicks off when necessary. I must do that to cope with this new reality, death facing me. Me facing death.
> (Butler & Rosenblum, 1991: 123)

As a whole, the book (Butler & Rosenblum, 1991) is a blend, in Frank's (2013) narrative terms of memoir and restitution. In the excerpts, Barbara's writing indicates a shift to living in an empty present (Davies, 1997) tinged with chaos. Sandy continues to reflect, as she does in much of the book, that she is living in the future, her story will not end with Barbara's death. While their account appears to be written in open awareness (Timmermans, 1994) of Barbara's approaching death, the quotations suggest that the awareness was more akin to conditional openness (Field & Copp, 1999). This mode reflects the transience of the emotional and cognitive responses by patients and their partner/carers to imminent death. Barbara also seems to have moved to the third of the four 'readiness to die' modes, "person not ready, body ready" (Copp, 1998: 388). In her study of hospice nursing perspectives of dying, Copp (1996) proposed a separation between the body and the self indicative of a person's readiness to die. Generally this was characterised as a shift from 'person not ready, body ready' to 'person ready, body ready' but she acknowledged a shift between any of the four modes was possible. Barbara senses her body signalling a readiness to die to which she must adjust and accept. Yet she lives a further eight months until Sandy writes "At exactly eleven-fifteen the next morning, Valentine's Day, you sent me in to the kitchen for some fresh water, smiling up at me with love. When I re-entered our room, just moments later, with herb tea and ice water, you were already dead" (Butler & Rosenblum, 1991: 170).

The many months between Barbara's observation that she is facing death and the actual event, suggest that the actual process of mind–body separation is longer than might be inferred from "the terminal phase ... when the dying person starts to withdraw from the outside world" (Copp, 1998: 385). Specifying the likely duration required for terminal care is a controversial but necessary topic in the planning of palliative care provision (Murray et al., 2005). I will limit discussion to this definition "the management of patients during their last few days or weeks or even months of life from a point at which it becomes clear that the patient is in a progressive state of decline" (Maltoni & Amadori, 2001: 449). However, the authors go on to amplify the weeks and months to up to a year when death can be expected to occur. The lay public may prefer this more prosaic definition "When you reach that place where you have been told – and you believe – that you are going to die within a certain amount of time: that is the Death Zone" (Gould, 2012: 119). Barbara described her sense of detachment which would seem to support Copp's (1998) suggestion of withdrawal over Gould's (2012) desire to accept medical wisdom.

In the second pair of excerpts, Marion describes a clinic visit:

> In the consulting room of the diabetes nurse Tom looks very sick. The lighting is aggressive and I see him clearly for the first time in days. Though bright, our house is nowhere as evenly lit as this ... we are both wearing the clothes we got up in not very long ago and Tom looks eroded and shabby around the edges. He is a big, dark garden rose blown out at the end of the season, a hybrid purple and black. His eyes are dulled. His hair is damp with sweat. His silhouette was always dynamic, strangely elastic and crisp for a large man, and kept its energy well. Now he seems loose, his flesh not kempt but wayward, no longer trimmed in tight by the body's pull. Forces other than gravity are at work. Gravity drags down while the cancer pushes out from the centre ...
>
> I observe him. Is he going to fall over? I wonder. He hasn't yet, but might at any point. Is he asleep? Will he be able to get out of the chair again? Getting out of the chair is a complex muscular action that his legs and forearms strain to do. He is a dying man. That is what he looks like. How long has his skin been this pale yellowish-grey? It's as pale as joiner's putty or porcelain unfired.
> *(Coutts, 2014: 182–3)*

It was difficult to identify appropriately concurrent entries from the two accounts as Marion's version is not always dated nor in temporal sequence. However, this extract from Tom's book is within a week or two of Marion's above:

> Things are very much lost. I can't really write at all, except very late, and very limitedly.
> At the moment it's only 7pm. I want to think about my article: about the beginning of this life.

It was exactly two years ago. This life began with my first fit. My immediate symptom was recognised as a brain tumour – with the very first operation – and the fact that my life wouldn't last very long.

My acceptance of death. My gratitude for medicine.

Though the future was always waiting.

And then, rather recently, there have been the growing problems with speech.

And it's very hard on the limbs.

(Lubbock, 2012: 140–1)

Marion writes as the artist she is, visually, rich with colour and detailed description. We see the crumpled, decaying rose slumped in the chair and sense her awareness of his dying now being too near to ignore. Tom's writing is one of the last entries he made before he lost the ability to read and write. With the help of Marion and friends, his essay was published in *The Observer*.[7] Four months later he died, the nature of his illness necessitating hospital and hospice care for the last two months. Marion's description of Tom's death comes slowly over a few pages with scattered interruptions from hospice life and visiting friends:

Tom is already elsewhere, gone on his own sometime in the last days. He glided so delicately out, his absence so continuous with his presence, with us and without us, that I didn't catch the moment and immediately it happened it had already gone and was behind me. So. Just me …

Stay, stay awhile, I whisper to the bed …

I want this death to happen because it is the end and I will finally rest. I don't want it to happen because it is the beginning and I will finally understand. We are together on the bed. It is familiar. Like how we were.

How precious, I tell him, we are here and I am seeing you off. I am sending you. My hand is in his hand. Go. I hum something, not anything. Go. I speak words, not anything. Go. I am not anything. Go. I am.

(Coutts, 2014: 289–91)

Both of the partner extracts, Sandy's and Marion's, describe life continuing, being lived as full as it could be in the circumstances. In practice, the dying person remains in their chosen place, their home or hospice home "This is a place he can die well with us around him. Suddenly, overnight, we are home" (Coutts, 2014: 265). In both partner accounts there is a steady stream of visitors: friends, family, colleagues, for Barbara the rabbi, and for Tom and Marion their three year old son. And there is open awareness of Barbara and Tom detaching, not always present to each occasion, drifting.

In both, albeit very different accounts, I sense much of my own experience of Jane's death. As partner/carer, even with the many forms and embodiments of support, an exhausted saturation point is reached. It is almost as if through the dying process the burden of the death act shifts from the dying person to their partner. One reaches their zenith with death and the other is released to a sorrowful nadir. Marion has it perfectly "I want this death to happen because it is the end and I will finally rest. I don't want it to happen because it is the beginning and I will finally understand" (Coutts, 2014: 290). Marion is with Tom as he dies but Sandy has been sent away for iced water by Barbara who dies before her return. I was asleep, lying beside Jane and believing the slightest movement or noise would wake me. Yet I felt ashamed, that I had failed her in some way by being asleep. Equally, I had the feeling that it was her choice, as with Barbara, it was something private that she wanted without my gaze.

The art and aesthetics of nursing

Having considered writing about illness I now want to return to the nature of aesthetic experience, first as a facet of nursing practice and then as expressed through the philosophical work of Schiller. In my efforts to understand my experience of Jane's illness and death, I first rejected the former nurse within me. My experience as a nurse and of training is briefly mentioned in the first chapter. But it has taken years of intense study and reconsidering my love–hate relationship with nursing, to appreciate as a return enhanced what being a nurse now means to me. Becoming a nurse was a rite of passage between the familiar, secular world of London in the mid-1970s and the sacred world of healing as practised in a major Scottish teaching hospital. The experience featured all three of van Gennep's (1960) phases or rites: separation, transition and incorporation. I was separated from my home, my family and my freedom by the requirement to live in the probationer nurses' home for the first six months of training. It was as if I had entered a religious order with its rules, regulations and uniform dress. It took three years to complete the transition from gauche novice to independent practitioner. This was an apprentice system where we learnt by imitation and knowledge acquisition (Carper, 1978), knowing not to question what we saw or were told. Obedience was necessary for organisational control (Fisher & Freshwater, 2014), both in the school of nursing and the hospital. Once qualified, we became 'staff nurses' and were reincorporated in the secular world where the ill needed our care with its special skills and knowledge. Yet this was also a time of transition for nursing as a profession, although what was being incorporated was more concerned with the secular than the sacred.

There is neither time nor space to enter into a detailed explanation of the professionalisation of nursing over the past forty years. However, it is worth noting that I had no sooner qualified when everything I held sacred about nursing was overturned by the demand for a scientific basis to its nature and management (Allen & Lyne, 2006). Florence Nightingale described nursing as an art that was mostly concerned with cleanliness and practical common sense, typically the work of women. Children grow up with the hand of their mother cooling their fevered brow or salving their scuffed knees. A strong sense of the caring mother figure was nursing's companion story. I had the added bonus of exciting stories from my mother of the hospital ward featuring glamorous nurses and amorous male doctors. While she portrayed a romanticised view of caring work it nevertheless held certain attractions, sounding both scary and exciting. She omitted to tell me the reality of what blood and gore really smell like, but her message was clear. I needed to earn my living, I was not bright enough to be a doctor, but nursing was a good alternative. It was only much later that I realised she was legitimating her own life choices. From an early age, I had been trained in the traditional art of nursing, the laying on of hands and caring for the sick. I graduated from plastic dolls to my younger siblings as I crafted my art. My childhood reading from my mother's collection was Pugh's *Practical Nursing* (1944) which details the qualities of a good nurse:

> To become a good nurse, a woman must possess intelligence, a good education, healthy physique, good manners, an even temper, a sympathetic temperament, and deft clever hands. To these she must add habits of observation, punctuality, obedience, cleanliness, a sense of proportion, and a capacity for and habit of accurate statement. Training can only strengthen these qualities and habits; it cannot produce them.
>
> (Pugh, 1944: 3)

Feminists may well pale at this specification, more so when they learn that it is unchanged from the original version of the text written by a physician and a matron from St Bartholomew's Hospital, London (Stewart & Cuff, 1899). The definition persisted unchanged to its final edition (Pugh, 1969). It depicts the archetypal nurse, unintentionally romanticised, instantly recognisable and symbolic of the reassuring care that a sick person might wish for themselves. There is an implied maturity to this prototype nurse. She is not a girl who will become a woman through her training, she arrives as a woman already educated and demure. To this I aspired; I could become this person if I successfully completed the rites of passage that constituted nurse training in the 1970s. What we learnt was procedural, task-oriented, a system of techniques that could be performed in many settings, not just in hospitals. It was practised on passive patients in the role of obedient recipients of these administrations. I was taught not to care as such but to give comfort by ensuring sheets were straight and crumb-free, pillows were plumped and artfully arranged, all seasoned with a light peppering of reassuring prattle. This was the art and craft of nursing. It follows that if nursing is considered to be an art there must be a connection with aesthetics but not necessarily as a philosophy of the beautiful.

I do not intend to provide an overview or an analysis of the evolutionary development of nursing over the last forty years save one aspect: the tension between nursing as an art and as a science. In an attempt to clarify and give value to the softer, less definable and evidential aspects of nursing, Carper proposed a model of nursing knowledge, derived from her doctoral research that recognised the scientific aspects of nursing as 'empirics' and the art of nursing as 'esthetics'[8] (Carper, 1978). The model is presented as four patterns of 'knowing' with the addition of personal knowledge in nursing and ethics as a moral component. In questioning the traditional, task-oriented and fragmented approach, an alternative, aesthetic pattern of nursing is proposed where "One gains knowledge of another person's singular, particular, felt experience through empathic acquaintance" (Carper, 1978: 17). This configuration centres on the relationship between the patient as an individual, and the nurse with a repertoire of special skills or aesthetic knowing based on the particular, not the universal. Carper's model stimulated much subsequent research into the theory and practice of nursing (for comprehensive appraisal see Wainwright, 2000 and Zander, 2007).

The arguments against nursing as an art form are as much to do with the concern for scientific rationality and recognition of nursing as a human science (Derbyshire, 1999) as they are concerned with aesthetic appreciation. The overtly feminist language used by some authors (Chinn, 1994; Chinn & Kramer, 2010) combined with a clearly arts-informed narrative as used, for example, by Gaydos (2006) may have undermined the essence of the argument. Examples of simple actions such as a nurse placing her hand on an anxious person's shoulder as reassurance (Chinn & Kramer, 2010), spending time with a patient (Gaydos, 2006), or creating a social space for an illness story to be told (Leight, 2001), may support the claim of an aesthetic quality to nursing. However, these examples could also be interpreted as empathic, "the capacity for participating in or vicariously experiencing another's feelings" (Carper, 1978: 17), which she contends is an important aspect of the aesthetic pattern of knowing in nursing. This connects with the earlier point in this chapter from Frank (2013) on the reciprocity of empathy. In a comparison between the writings of Florence Nightingale and Carper's model (Clements & Averill, 2006) there is evidence of the empathic role of the nurse:

> Nightingale clearly discussed the necessary *presence* of the nurse with the client, as well as interpersonal interface and communication, as a pathway to knowing. She validated that knowing about the client is experiential, as well as shared. In essence, for a nurse to be empathetic toward a client, she or he must be fully present, at that moment, sharing the experience and what it means to both the nurse and the client at the time. Aesthetic knowing is clearly bound by consciousness, proximity, and human interchange at various levels.
>
> *(Clements & Averill, 2006: 270, original emphasis)*

The challenge in nursing and therefore for nurses, has always been to help the sick to feel better, to provide comfort and through compassion, to alleviate their suffering (Bouchal, 2007). The ability to give this care is both inherent, as a basic genderless, human response, and in the skills taught. The nursing profession has striven to make the necessary knowledge and expertise explicit, changing nurse education from the apprenticeship model of accepted practice to an academic discipline founded on research evidence. My fascination with the difference between nurses as they perform their daily customs and rituals was rekindled when Jane was ill. I had a front row seat in the chemo unit or the day ward. Why did Jane, and by extension I, prefer some nurses to others? Was it just personality or was there something more to the nature of their performance and was this somehow aesthetic? In simple terms, some nurses were easier than others, made more time for reassuring chat or were highly efficient in their work. Perhaps this can be explained by "With aesthetic knowledge, the nurse expresses the artistic nature of nursing care by appreciating the act of caring for individuals" (Siles-Gonzalez & Solano-Ruiz, 2015: 5). The implication being that some nurses are more in touch or comfortable with their own feelings when caring for others.

When practising as a nurse, I generally felt uncomfortable with myself and certainly was not in touch with my feelings. I often felt powerless in the presence of overwhelming trauma, illness and suffering. I could see how much hurt and pain there was but beyond performing the tasks expected of me as a nurse, I could not engage empathetically with the patient. On occasion, this failing was perceived by more senior nurses who questioned my ability to care and to be a competent nurse. Part of my earlier interest in nursing research was to try and understand what constituted this aspect of nursing that I failed to understand. I avoided nursing contexts that would require longer relationships with patients, preferring accident and emergency or the operating theatre. When I did become a charge nurse in an acute medical ward where patient stays were longer, I could distance myself from close contact through my managerial role. When Jane was ill, I was trapped in close proximity to someone who needed my care. Although much of the time during the Illness Period I was busy *doing* all aspects of running the household and caring for Jane, I came to realise that *being* near was what I had hitherto failed to understand.

The nature of aesthetic experience

Having explored the aesthetic aspects of nursing practice, I now want to consider the nature of aesthetic experience, initially from the perspective of someone who is dying. Jane realised that "you will lose your hair" (Blog post, 'Silver Linings', day 45) and the transformation by the disease of her lithesome body into a bloated caricature was an intense suffering for both of us. How might any of this be remotely concerned with aesthetics, the appreciation of the beautiful? I will argue that it is in the stark reality of facing death that a perceptual clarity emerges enabling the transcendence of the phenomenal to the noumenal.[9] Sensations are heightened as their experience returns to the intellect in a process of enhancement and mediation. Explanations of aesthetic experience are invariably traced back to Kant despite the fact that his definition of the pleasurable observation of an object was by implication "the type of experience we have of those objects which we declare beautiful, and on which experiences our particular judgments of taste can be founded" (Neville, 1974: 193). A more recent sociological interpretation of Kant suggests that the aesthetic experience of cultural objects is characterised by the "free play of cognitive and numinous experience unstructured by concepts" (Battani, 2011: 1) and that "the form of the experience is dictated as much by cognitive structure as it is by social structure" (Battani, 2011: 12). Similarly, and in relation to arts-based research, the impediment to the Kantian interpretation of aesthetic experience which confines it to fine art is challenged (Jagodzinski & Wallin, 2013). Nevertheless, the emphasis continues to be in relation to the making and perception of art and its objects. A more spiritual view takes into account both the mystical aspects of the aesthetic alluded to by the philosopher William James and the relevance of nature, concluding with the suggestion that the varieties of aesthetic experience act as a gateway to "cosmic consciousness" (Jones, 2014). Yet aesthetic experience has an embodied and therefore phenomenological dimension to its cognitive perception (Joy & Sherry, 2003; Carel, 2011) as well as any spiritual dimension.

The complex nature and difficulty in determining a precise, contemporary definition for aesthetic experience[10] now questions its value and existence (Tomlin, 2010). Generally, it is described as an engagement with art or nature as a deeply moving piece of music, an exquisite painting or a beautiful landscape. In this sense, aesthetic experience "is precious and of fundamental value to human beings" (Tomlin, 2010: 1). In a collection of essays (Shusterman & Tomlin, 2010) resulting from a conference on the value of aesthetic experience, there is no unified definition but a range of interpretations. Renewed consideration of aesthetic experience could have the "potential to positively transform oneself, our fellow sentient beings and our environment" (Tomlin, 2010: 11). Again, exigency here negates a detailed appraisal of the arguments but Shusterman's contribution to the debate, particularly his examination of the end of aesthetic experience (Shusterman, 1997, 2006) and his concept of somaesthetics (Shusterman, 1999; 2011), are noteworthy. Briefly, Shusterman argues that the decline of aesthetic experience in terms of its philosophical Anglo-American traditions has resulted from the emergence of theoretical tensions between four definitional dimensions: evaluative, phenomenological, semantic and demarcational (Shusterman, 1997: 30). Viewed in this way aesthetic experience is valuable and enjoyable, vividly felt, meaningful and generally distinctive as art. It has become a state where the "transformational notion of aesthetic experience has been gradually replaced by a purely descriptive, semantic one whose chief purpose is to explain and this supports the established demarcation of art from other domains" (Shusterman, 1997: 32).

In asserting that the body has a complex role in aesthetic experience, the notion of somaesthetics has been proposed as "essentially concerned with human flourishing by focusing on improving the use of one's embodied self and one's somatic experience" (Shusterman, 2011: 323). The concept was derived both from Shusterman's own work in aesthetics and his embrace of eastern esoteric traditions. The term soma in this context is concerned with the inner or felt experience of the body and not its outward appearance (Arnold, 2005). Dance exemplifies somaesthetics where the soma conceived in "the form of its physical skills, senses and pleasures plays no less a part in the living of a full life than conceptual understanding and the imaginative use of language" (Arnold, 2005: 48). To summarise, the phenomenological nature of aesthetic experience implies a sensate focus on an object as an experience felt in a particular way. If aesthetic experience is about something, it must have some dimension of meaning (Shusterman, 2006). In an echo of Heidegger's (1977) concern regarding purely instrumental definitions of technology that disregard its essence, Shusterman argues that the value of aesthetic experience is all but lost to information technology as our "affective capacities wear thin" (Shusterman, 1997: 39). Then he reminds us of the "illustrious tradition of exploring aesthetics as a key to ethics and the art of living" (Shusterman, 1999: 308) which he finds exemplified in Schiller's *Aesthetic Letters*, to which I will now return.

Schiller's aesthetic education

Earlier I outlined the essential argument of Schiller's *Aesthetic Letters* and their precursor, the *Kallias Letters*. In this context there are two particular points to highlight from the latter, first to "interpret Schiller properly requires us both to recognize the distinction of meanings and to hold them at the same time together in a reciprocally illuminating unity" (Schindler, 2008: 89). And as I described in the first chapter, this necessitates an appreciation of *Gestalt* as both an understanding of not just the inner idea of something as matter, concretion, and organisation as a whole, but also its outward appearance. In this respect, Goethe's influence on Schiller is acknowledged (Bishop, 2008; Schindler, 2008), but *form* in the context of aesthetics, should always being prefixed by 'living'.[11] The complex metaphysical point being made is that *form* offers a semblance of life but it also articulates life as felt. It was this *felt life* that both Goethe and Schiller found to be true of all art. To further explain the point, something can be recognised as being beautiful without being first understood, but then as understanding develops, appreciation deepens. This is "the 'both/and' character of form" (Schindler, 2008: 90) as presented by Schiller. The second relevant point from the *Kallias Letters*, concerns Schiller's interpretation of freedom as an intuitive action devoid of ulterior motive:

> An action is morally beautiful, then, if on the one hand it is the fulfilment of a duty that is 'imposed,' so to speak, as an absolute necessity, and, on the other hand, it occurs as if it springs directly from the inner being of the agent as a wholly spontaneous act. That is to say, it comes simultaneously from without and from within.
>
> (Schindler, 2008: 93)

This is not simply the mechanistic performance of a task but an action that arises spontaneously from an inner sense of both moral duty and technical ability. On this basis, I suggest that with regard to nursing, a nurse may act routinely and quite correctly but perhaps lacks a sense of what might be described as 'nurseness' or even 'careness'. This means a nurse with an inner sense of Schillerian freedom acts intuitively, as if without conscious thought, and is therefore more 'physically present' (Schindler, 2008: 92). In turn, this speaks to the presence of the nurse as an aesthetic knowledge that is "clearly bound by consciousness, proximity, and human interchange at various levels" (Clements & Averill, 2006: 270). I had a sense of this, as an inner knowing, when caring for Jane, a feeling that had eluded me when I actually worked as a nurse. This might also be interpreted as my recognition of how "empathic imagination is a central faculty for integrating the head, hand and heart" (Galvin & Todres, 2007: 42).

The justification for this attention to Schiller's interpretation of aesthetics is twofold. First, although I know Jane understood these subtle dualisms in a particular way, I cannot provide much in the way of actual evidence beyond citing her work written twenty years previously. I realised that I had noticed something subtle in her demeanour during her illness. She makes little reference to it in the blog during her illness but there was something in the way she carried herself, an almost tragic serenity. At the time, this was generally perceived by friends and family as courage, stoicism and bravery. While these characteristics were true, what I saw was her physical suffering counter-balanced by a sense of inner calm. This is the dance between outer discomfort and inner peace, between seeing me as her healthy, living partner while she herself is dying. She knew, from her studies of both Schiller and Goethe, that this was unity, a holistic way of being. Through this study I can now interpret this as the manifestation of the phenomena of her illness and the noumenal rationalisation of her prognosis transcended through aesthetic experience. That said, I am also aware that a claim is being made that the methodological process of Jane's doctoral work led to a personal transformation of her own beliefs and will now provide some illustrations from the material gathered in the course of the study in its support.

In the context of living with life-limiting illness, pleasurable feelings resulting from an aesthetic experience have the potential to transcend "Even momentary wholeness gives us renewed reserves of psychic energy with which to meet the moral challenges of our lives and a refined sensibility to apply in our dealings with the world" (Sharpe, 1991: 160). A simple example from Jane illustrates this point "I think I sometimes see things more intensely now – I thought eiders were black and white birds, I'd never really noticed that they have pinkish chests, and the most beautiful blue-green hue to their cheeks" (Blog post 'Catching Up: Plants, Gardens, Cars and Other Things', day 291). Similarly, the playwright Dennis Potter describes the plum tree he can see from his window as he writes "I see it is the whitest, frothiest, blossomest blossom that there ever could be" (Bragg, 2007). Viktor Frankl in his memoir of concentration camp survival, recalls a dying woman being sustained by the view from her window where "she could see just one branch of a chestnut tree, and on the branch were two blossoms … [she talked to the tree and the tree replied] 'I am here – I am here – I am life, eternal life'" (Frankl, 2004: 78). All three accounts are recollections of seeing the dynamic nature of life and not the static artifice of the arts.

A connection can be made from aesthetic experience and its relationship to binary synthesis through Goethe's scientific philosophy to phenomenology. For Goethe aesthetic experience is "the indirect way by means of which ('subjective') Idea and ('objective') Experience converge" (Stephenson, 2005: 567, original emphasis). This interpretation is cognate with the ideas Schiller develops in *Letters 6 to 22*:

> Goethe, like Schiller, distinguished not only between different modalities of the imagination, but also between those of aesthetic experience. The aesthetic

also operates in three different modalities: there is the "subordinate" role that Schiller envisages for the aesthetic as the prime matter, as it were, on which the intellect goes to work in order to produce concepts and theory; there is the "co-ordinate" role as direct object of enjoyment; and there is its "super-ordinate" role in gracious living.

(Stephenson, 2005: 567 fn5)

For example, if I look at a red rose growing in my garden I see it as a direct object subordinated through the conceptual lens of botanical art (in which I have some training) and experience a certain pleasure in the rose's appearance. The aesthetic deepens as I see the rose's red colour as an outward expression of its internal meaning or redness (Schindler, 2008). It is in this fundamental interplay that we sense the rhythmic patterns of the real world as "tension, intensity, and resolution" (Stephenson, 2005: 568). Furthermore:

> Thinking and doing, breathing in and breathing out, moving backwards and moving forwards, question and answer: pairs of opposites which make sense only in relation to one another, which function fully only in coordination ... Binary synthesis is descriptive of the process of existence rather than prescriptive of the process of logic. The oppositions in a binary synthesis function truly only together, but they remain distinct: either or both of the fundamental polarities appears enhanced through reciprocal, subordinating interaction with the other.

(Plenderleith, 1993: 298)

And it is in Jane's own words that there is a sense of the natural rhythm of life, the ebb and flow of living and dying. The red rose will wilt, shedding its petals on the ground where they will gradually decompose and feed the bush itself. For all their complex abstractions, both Schiller and Goethe are describing natural processes of life, complete with an asymmetrical co-ordination of opposites. For, in Goethe's world "there are no perfect Forms; only beautifully-formed imperfections" (Stephenson, 2005: 569). I believe it was in this sense of nature's beautiful imperfections that Jane understood her cancer "My body has done this to itself" (Blog post, 'A Different Mindset', day 98). There is also a connection between Goethean science and human geography that informs the understanding of place (Seamon, 1979; Brook, 1998; Cameron, 2005). This links to the earlier finding[12] regarding the embodied feeling of being at home and unhomelikeness (Svenaeus, 2003).

Being in a human world

The link between Goethe's scientific writing and interpretations of place is through phenomenology to humanistic geography, a discipline that has a particular interest in a different way of looking at the human inhabited world (Seamon, 1979). Although Goethe's interest was in the experiential study of phenomena as they appear in nature, the philosophical discipline of *phenomenology* did not emerge until the twentieth century with the conceptual language of Edmund Husserl (Seamon, 1998). His purpose in developing phenomenology was to find a method for investigating the lifeworld which "places the problematic of human consciousness and its world-constitution at the center of phenomenological inquiry" (Simms, 2005: 171). Unsurprisingly, phenomenology has become a significant approach in the study of human experience in health and illness, particularly nursing (Dowling, 2007) and includes iterations through such luminaries as Heidegger, Merleau-Ponty and Gadamer (Wojnar & Swanson, 2007).

The particular aspect of humanistic geography that relates to this study is the relationship people have with the places in their lifeworld, defined as "the culturally defined spatiotemporal setting or horizon of everyday life" (Buttimer, 1976: 277). While many factors may disrupt our relationship with particular locations such as home or work place, ill health can be an additional existential disturbance to spatial life. The co-ordinated movements of daily life such as washing, cooking or knitting form habitual routines in space and time, termed as "place ballets" (Seamon, 1979: 56). The movements are choreographed and performed by the person as they negotiate their way through the places and routines of daily life. The familiarity of this dance changes as new places require accommodation; this can be both exhilarating and challenging. On occasion the bustle of street life may appear attractive after a period of isolation but the sterile uniformity of a busy hospital corridor may arouse feelings of *dis-ease*. The latter can be understood as 'placelessness' which describes both "an environment without significant places and the underlying attitude which does not acknowledge significance in places" (Relph, 1976: 143).

Hospitals cause a sense of placelessness for their patients. Even when some personal ephemera are permitted, the actual bed space occupied may be frequently changed by service pressures. A precious view from a window may be lost when a bed is turned to face another direction; a preferred seat in a day care unit may not be available. These may seem trivial, incidental examples but I suggest that the experiential significance of place in health care environments is poorly understood and generally ignored for expediency. The discussion of place would be incomplete without attention to the place most people feel at ease, their home. Previously I have raised the sense of displacement and discomfort that can arise from not feeling 'at-home'. In a broader sense, this is both a place of rest and can refer to "any situation in which the person or an object with which he or she has contact is relatively fixed in place and space for a longer or shorter period of time" (Seamon, 1979: 69). So it could be, for example, a place of work, medical treatment or even a café. However, it is the dwelling place or home that is the spatial centre of 'at-homeness':

> the usually unnoticed, taken-for-granted situation of being comfortable in and familiar with the everyday world in which one lives and outside of which one is 'visiting', 'in transit', 'not at home', 'out of place' or 'travelling'.
>
> *(Seamon, 1979: 70)*

At-homeness is manifest in feelings of rootedness, appropriation, regeneration, at-easeness and warmth (Seamon, 1979: 87). In addition to these aspects, the sense of at-homeness is further enhanced by Heidegger's notion of dwelling in the sense of sparing and preserving (Seamon, 1979: 92). Environmental awareness is an indicator of this, where dwelling with a care-taking role finds "the free sphere that safeguards each thing in its essence" (Heidegger, 1993: 351). It follows that an individual might have heightened awareness but feel quite alien to their surroundings, not at one with their world. For example a patient newly admitted to hospital and sitting bolt upright in bed, may be intensely aware of their surroundings yet appear oblivious as they struggle to cope with the new environment.

A more recent although not directly related work recognises that "Goethean research demonstrates that each living creature has a unique manner of presence in the world" (Seamon, 2005: 98). As humans this presence is how we appear, behave, live and experience the world. Nevertheless, what Seamon describes as heightened contact is in fact an excellent foundational definition of aesthetic experience, notwithstanding the earlier remarks regarding such definitions. In light of this, I suggest that in addition to the phenomenal and noumenal aspects of aesthetic experience, there is also context. This addition can then account for not having an aesthetic experience when someone alongside does, as in the case of personal preferences for art, music and vistas. Or in an embodied context between being well and being ill, particularly for those who are dying. It is in this context that I now define aesthetic experience as *feeling a serenity of mood, a vividness of presence and a heightened self awareness*. In short, a sense of oneness which is recognisable by its intensity and striking presence. There is also a strong, albeit unintentional, connection to the earlier[13] definition of the features of aesthetic experience from Wilkinson and Willoughby, as "sensibility refined, feeling quickened, imagination enriched, and understanding enlarged".[14] I make no apology for repeating the quotation nor this example from Jane "I think I sometimes see things more intensely now – I thought eiders were black and white birds, I'd never really noticed that they have pinkish chests, and the most beautiful blue-green hue to their cheeks" (Blog post 'Catching Up: Plants, Gardens, Cars and Other Things', day 291). I remember the scene on the beach in North Berwick as the sun was setting and the eider ducks were coming home to settle for the night. There was an intensity to the light, it was on my birthday in February and their breeding plumage was indeed vivid. In that moment her dying and my living were irrelevant; we were both present watching the bobbing ducks with divine pleasure. Sometimes an aesthetic experience can be shared, especially in the context of two people who share a deep, emotional relationship.

Sociability and communitas

There is a further aspect of aesthetic experience to which I have previously alluded regarding human companionship. It touches on the nature of the caring relationship in both an individual and a wider sense; as the interaction between a nurse and her patient or between the patient and her companions. The German sociologist Georg Simmel (1858–1918) had a lifelong interest in Kant and Goethe (Lee & Silver, 2013). Throughout his life he sought connections between sociology and aesthetics (Fuente, 2008) which he came to describe as sociability, "the play-form of association [which] is related to the content-determined concreteness of association as art is related to reality" (Simmel, 1949: 255). The reciprocal and relational nature of the interaction is characterised by the principle that "the pleasure of the individual is always contingent upon the joy of others" (Simmel, 1949: 257). Others have noted the connection to Schiller's aesthetics (Fuente, 2008; Lee & Silver, 2013) but not that the play-form is a drive "which presses toward this form of existence and often only later calls forth that objective content which carries the particular association along" (Simmel, 1949: 255). This could also be interpreted in Schiller's terms of human drives where the play-form (play-drive) emerges through the association with existential form (form-drive) which is then organised by the 'objective content' (material-drive). In other words, there is "more to his account of the aesthetics of social life than the insight that form separates art, or for that matter any type of aesthetic experience, from the rest of life" (Fuente, 2008: 353).

In this context, the most relevant aspect of Simmel's work which exemplifies the aesthetics of social life, is his sociability of the meal (Simmel, 1997). His argument starts from the premise that eating and drinking are the thing people have in common. From this he then draws his interpretation of the meal as a sociological matter that "arranges itself in a more aesthetic, stylized and supra-individually regulated form" (Simmel, 1997: 131). The meal is the basis for the convergence of aesthetic and social form through its processes of social bonding (Fuente, 2008). As an aesthetic experience eating is entirely individual, we cannot eat the same food but the same sounds and images can be enjoyed. For Simmel as a sociological structure it "attains a synthesis of individuality and commonality rare even among the cultivated arts" (Fuente, 2008: 358). It was this form of aesthetic experience that was the most powerful for Jane and she recounts many shared meals in the blog. Confidentiality negates much quotation but this extract is illustrative:

> a work colleague came for lunch. We had a lovely, warm, intimate and insightful conversation, touching on a wide variety of topics, from the state of technology-enhanced learning in UK higher education to body donation. As [he] said, no-one could accuse us of small talk.
> *(Blog post 'Friends and Family', day 307)*

While at this late stage in her illness, Jane was unable to actually eat much, she could fully participate in the conviviality:

> The fact that we must eat is a fact of life situated so primitively and elementarily in the development of our life-values that it is unquestionably shared by each individual with every other one. This is precisely what makes gathering together for a shared meal possible in the first place, and the

transcendence of the mere naturalism of eating develops out of the socialization mediated in this way.

(Simmel, 1997: 135)

However, Simmel gave his paper on the sociability of the meal to the first meeting of the German Sociological Society in 1910, at a time which goes some way to explain his class bias "Compared with the image of someone eating in a farm house or at a workers' festival, a dinner in educated circles appears to be completely schematized and regulated" (Simmel, 1997: 132). Nevertheless he uses the orderly principles of aesthetics to illustrate how behaviour during the meal is regulated as people take turns to serve themselves. Even when someone is dying, their participation in the very basic orderly structure of a shared meal acts as a balance to the otherwise disruptive chaos of their illness. Jane's blog posts are punctuated with food enjoyed as is Coutts' (2014) memoir of her dying husband with its frequent lists of food and appetising descriptions of food gifts. More poignant is the flask of special fish soup she brings her husband in the hospice "Talking to the chef I have the urge to tell him who the soup is for, as if to stress to him how much it means. But I don't say anything ... I do the errand and hurry back. He eats three teaspoons before he stops" (Coutts, 2014: 284).

The importance of the meal in the context of the dying can be further emphasised by reading it as part of rite-of-passage ritual. Simmel contrasts world religions and "the cults of antiquity [who gather] together for the sacrificial meal" (Simmel, 1997: 130). For the dying person this may be an opportunity for what Victor Turner terms spontaneous communitas, a relationship that "appears to flourish best in spontaneously liminal situations – phases betwixt and between states where social-structural role-playing is dominant, and especially between status equals" (Turner, 1969: 138). Spontaneous communitas is akin to what hippies might have called "a happening" (Turner, 1969: 132), which could be described as the impromptu congregation of people to engage in the mutual appreciation of each other's company. Following his death, Turner's wife Edith continued to explore his ideas about ritual, rites of passage and his own term, communitas. She describes the connection he found "between the joy of communitas and rites of passage [as] moments of change freed from the structures of life" (Turner, 2012: 2). It can appear unexpectedly and it "often comes in the direst moments of the life of a person" (Turner, 2012: 2). In Jane's liminal, threshold state between living and dying, and having asserted her right to die at home, it becomes a sacred place. Here she can continue to participate in the ritual of shared meals with friends and family. There may be exquisite moments of intersection and alignment between the people attending, the sacred place of home and particular sensations: sights, sounds, smells, touches and tastes. These are the aesthetic experiences of dying, the mysterious, fleeting observations that those who are not dying might make:

> This evening we have a little party. A small group come for wine and songs. Tom knows the friends who come this evening. To each one's touch and

greeting he utters a different sound but his eyes are closed. Only when he hears the voice of Ev and his homecoming does he open them. I see this. I am the only one who does. I am so very lucky. I see that look.

(Coutts, 2014: 284)

Intuitively we know those moments, yet I doubt they can be collectively studied in any formal sense. While it is true that pleasure is not a necessary condition for aesthetic experience (Carroll, 2002), there may well be a bittersweet quality or an element of pathos to aesthetic experiences in the context of dying. But these are the precious moments in the memories of those who live on after the death of a loved one "[Jane's youngest sister] would come through in a heartbeat if I asked her to, but is busy with the hum of her life and anyway I agree with her that she'd prefer to remember me on the beach at St Andrews" (Blog post, 'So Much Love', day 330).

Coming home to Heidegger

I now want to explore how a sense of *at-homeness* was manifest for Jane and in light of her own interpretation of its significance for her as she described in Chapter 2: Prequel. As her illness progressed, difficult symptoms like ascites appeared, necessitating further encounters with hospital services. During these physical separations from the place where Jane was most at ease, I tried to maintain a sense of what I now understand as at-homeness. It was the little things: bringing her food, a scented hanky and a small basket of essentials (tissues, lip salve, glasses, pen, notebook, a dog knitted by my sister). She liked her bed to be beside a window with a view or at least a vista of somewhere else. So whether it was in the hospital or the hospice, she had the makings of home with an affordance of well-being.

Galvin and Todres have developed a conceptual framework of existential well-being in health care centred on the unity of dwelling-mobility (Todres & Galvin, 2010; Galvin & Todres, 2011a). Their theory is derived from Heidegger's ontological conceptualisation of homecoming (Todres & Galvin, 2010) where dwelling-mobility "is both 'the adventure' of being called into existential possibilities as well as 'the being at home with' what has been given. It carries with it a sense of rootedness and flow, peace and possibility" (Galvin & Todres, 2011a: 2). The authors acknowledge that while there are different interpretations of Heidegger, particularly as his work changed over time, they have found Mugerauer's (2008) analysis to be both accessible and consistent. It is worth noting that Heidegger's lifetime (1889–1976) spanned one of the most simultaneously innovative and destructive periods in human history. The effect not least of the atomic age has been attributed in his later writing to his interest in technology (Mugerauer, 2008). Heidegger argued that our addiction to the ease and flexibility of technological devices would determine our experience of everything in terms of its ease and flexibility (Dreyfus & Wrathall, 2004).

Heidegger is recognised as being difficult to understand and interpret not least because of his complicated use of language[15] (Dreyfus & Wrathall, 2004;

Mugerauer, 2008). In his desire to break with philosophical traditions he was both provocative in style and had a preference for neologisms. Language games are not without precedent in this study as the earlier discussions on aesthetic discourse[16] have illustrated. Direct connections between Goethe and/or Schiller and Heidegger are not obvious. Links to Goethe's colour theory and also to his conception of subject–object relations,[17] can be found in Heidegger's essay on 'Science and Reflection' (1977: 155). In the essay[18] and some of Heidegger's other writing there does seem to be a certain similarity, possibly an interpellation, reminiscent of both binary synthesis and the *Urphenomenon*. In addition, like Schiller, Heidegger employed a threefold pattern to his work: though not confined to a single text, it extended across his entire corpus (Mugerauer, 2008). To investigate what it means to be human, the conventional approach would be to either focus on the subjective, internal dimensions of life or the objective, external world. Like Goethe, Heidegger rejected this divide and wanted a way to see the human being and the world, not as separate but together (Mugerauer, 2008).

In *Being and Time* (1996), the text for which Heidegger is best known, he embarks upon an ambitious project to discover the meaning of being (Dreyfus & Wrathall, 2004). In fact, the book is the groundwork for his subsequent theories spanning his lifetime. A novel interpretation of much of Heidegger's corpus contends that his work is centred on the dynamic of "homelessness-homecoming-home" (Mugerauer, 2008: 17). Hölderlin, a contemporary and acquaintance of both Goethe and Schiller, and his poem, 'Homecoming' (Heidegger, 2000) was particularly influential for Heidegger. At first the poem appears to be about a joyful return home, but it was the last stanza that caught his attention where the word 'care' "suggests nothing of the joyful mood of someone who returns home care-free" (Heidegger, 2000: 32). In the poem he sets out an "ur-phenomenology of homecoming" (Mugerauer, 2008: 17). Through his comparative analysis of Heidegger and Hölderlin's poem, Mugerauer (2008: 17, my emphasis) has identified six phases to the phenomenon of homecoming:

1. initial being at home (even though not at home there)
2. *homelessness* or wandering in the foreign
3. turning towards home
4. a moment of *homecoming* or arrival
5. learning to become at home
6. abiding or dwelling near the primal source, the *home*

There is a binary synthesis between *homelessness* and *homecoming*, a return enhanced from wandering in foreign places to coming home, content to abide. Heidegger wrestles with the same dilemma as Goethe: how to re-present the complexities of a primal phenomena in discursive language. For both, the solution is poetry where Goethe finds "The presence of the Urphenomenon must be felt in its representation. Poetry is a re-symbolization of a primary symbolic event" (Stephenson, 2005: 573). And Heidegger in his later work develops a deeper and "*originary manner of thinking and saying* with which to *recover* ... the relationship of *poetizing language and the world*, and the focal phenomena of *dwelling, region, building* (Mugerauer, 2008: 11, original emphasis). Another way in which Heidegger practices his 'originary manner of thinking' is found in "meditative thinking [where there is] non-representational meanings that are thinking's proper analogue to poetry and mysticism" (Mugerauer, 2008: 12). However, although we are all capable of this kind of thinking, it lies dormant within us and needs to be awoken in order "to notice, to observe, to ponder, to awaken an awareness of what is actually taking place around us and in us" (Pezze, 2006: 100).

This thinking with heightened awareness and through poetry provides a connection to the kind of thinking necessary to appreciate and perceive the *Urphenomenon*. Heidegger does make the occasional specific reference to the *Urphenomenon*[19] as, for example "Not-being-at-home must be conceived existentially and ontologically as the more primordial phenomenon" (Heidegger, 1996: 177). But he frequently employs phenomenologically reduced terms (Sheehan, 2004) when, for example, he states "Being★ is the most 'universal' concept [as a footnote: ★the being, beingness]" (Heidegger, 1996: 2). In other words meaning becomes 'meaningfulness', a technique that is cognate with the earlier explanation[20] of red and 'redness', which is Schiller's both/and aesthetic form (Schindler, 2008). In phrases such as "Being is found in thatness and whatness, reality, the objective presence of things" (Heidegger, 1996: 5), what he is really trying to say, as he did in later work, is that it "is language that tells us about the essence of a thing" (Heidegger, 1993: 348). This claim is supported by the idea that category membership is a question of degree and not simply yes or no (Lakoff, 1973). For example in a "hierarchy of birdiness" (Lakoff, 1973: 459), a robin will have a higher position than a chicken or a bat. So birdiness is the extent to which the 'bird' matches its ideal type and in this sense can be interpreted in a manner similar to the *Urphenomenon*. What Heidegger seeks to achieve in what might be perceived as obfuscation, is the opposite. He wants to take us back to the earliest meaning of words which was why he was drawn to the poetry of Hölderlin and also mixes accepted meanings with neologisms.

Of the many words with which he played, there are two that I wish to explore in a little more detail. Neither word has an analogous variant in English, but approximations are given for each with references to fuller discussions. The first is *Gegnet* or 'abiding expanse' (Pezze, 2006) and the second is the previously mentioned[21] *Heimat*, which is somewhere between home and homeland but means neither (Hammermeister, 2000). For Heidegger, Heimat includes both "a linguistic and a regional aspect that in turn are mediated in dialect" (Hammermeister, 2000: 314). In this sense, dialect acts as an echo to an earlier language now lost to mankind. In addition to the sense of landscape and language, in the poetry of Hölderlin, there is both an "attempt to prepare for a reawakening sense of return to Heimat" (Hammermeister, 2000: 318). The idea of regionality is extended with *Gegnet*, an old form of the German word *Gegend* or region. Heidegger uses the older form to invoke a sense of "an enchanted region where everything belonging there returns to that in which it rests ... the region of all regions" (Pezze, 2006:

106). There is a sense of a hazy, distant horizon, somewhere in the future yet in full awareness of the past. This could also be understood as a return enhanced, not necessarily to a physical place but to the spirit of the sense evoked by remembering the place.

The aesthetic experience of dying

I now want to briefly consider the aesthetic in relation to landscape and the wider sense of geography. Extending the role of place in the lifeworld (Seamon, 1979) reveals it may also be a locale for aesthetic experience and as a place of healing, a therapeutic landscape (Gesler, 1992). However the therapeutic landscape is more "a geographic metaphor for aiding in the understanding of how the healing process works itself out in places" (Gesler, 1992: 743). Yet, using the already vague term landscape in this way is perhaps to 'stretch' (Brook, 2013) it too far. It is important to recognise that the concept of landscape needs to be understood as being 'lived in' and not simply 'viewed' (Brook, 2013: 109). While conventionally landscape may be romanticised as a picturesque panorama, as an aesthetic experience it requires engagement through an embodied whole "the fact that the landscape speaks to all our senses, and particularly the kinaesthetic sense, means that just to view it would be not only to miss the richness of the landscape experience but also to fail to become part of that aesthetic field" (Brook, 2013: 113). In this sense, our interaction with landscape could be considered a somaesthetic experience.

Jane had a strong sense of being Scottish, of being from a particular place with a distinctive landscape and a language that is more than a dialect of English. Two examples serve to illustrate this Scottishness in light of the discussion above. The first is a further interpretation of dwelling "*Wohnen* means to reside or stay, to dwell at peace, to be content; it is related to words that mean to grow accustomed to, or feel at home in, a place" (Heidegger, 1993: 345, translator's note). In Scots, 'stey' is more than dwell or reside, it is to "make one's home" (Robinson, 1985: 670). To me this suggests a certain flexibility or perhaps an ability to make oneself at home in changed circumstances. That is not to ignore the strong pull towards the homeland, but does imply an inner sense of a belonging that is portable. The second point is about the last books Jane read before she died: Lewis Grassic Gibbon's trilogy *A Scots Quair* (Gibbon, 2006). The stories tell in Scots, of the light, the land, and the language; Jane summarises the story:

> It's the move from rural village small-holding through the pusillanimity of the town to industrial unrest and economic depression in the city, from pastoral idyll through civic tensions to social disintegration, that makes the later works a more difficult read. But the parallels, echoes and progressions between the three works make it clear that these are not separate books, they are three integral and inter-related parts of the same whole.
>
> *(Blog post, 'Parallels, Echoes and Progression', day 240)*

It is not clear if the central character, Chris Guthrie, dies at the end but the following extracts from the final pages speaks to both *Gegnet* and to *Heimat* as the *Urphenomenon* of homecoming:

> Crowned with mists, Bennachie was walking into the night: and Chris moved and sat with her knees hand-clasped, looking far on that world across the plain and the day that did not die there but went east, on and on, over all the world till the morning came, the unending morning somewhere on the world. (671)
>
> Time she went home herself. But she still sat on as one by one the lights went out and the rain came, beating the stones about her, and falling all that night while she still sat there, presently feeling no longer the touch of the rain or hearing the sound of the lapwings going by.
>
> (Gibbon, 2006: 672)

I have come to realise that what this study does, amongst many other things, is to describe a story of coming home; to abide not just near to the primal source but at its heart, home. The study is also a validation of the Dwelling–Mobility lattice of well-being (Galvin & Todres, 2011b) as a 'place ballet' of aesthetic experiences. Earlier in this chapter the six phases of the phenomena of homecoming drawn from Heidegger's synthesis of Hölderlin's poetry were listed. Goethe often used poetry in his scientific writing when he felt discursive language had reached its limit as "Aesthetic experience can be represented only by aesthetic experience" (Stephenson, 2005: 573). Although the extract from *A Scots Quair* is prose, it has a strong poetic quality that could be presented as a poem; for me it represents the aesthetic experience of homecoming. Returning, enhanced, to the six phases they can stand for a lifetime or a time in a life when something momentous occurred. Taking the version articulated by Hölderlin then elucidated by Heidegger as the poetic journey (Mugerauer, 2008: 119), I have added (shown in emphasis) the phases of Jane's journey, as recounted in Chapters 4 to 6:

1. an initial being at home that is not yet a being at home; at the beginning the poetic spirit is not at home in its own house   *Wondering*
2. homelessness or wandering in the foreign and unhomely   *Finding, Planning, Treating*
3. a turning point – back towards home – return home   *Turning*
4. a moment of homecoming or arrival   *Living*
5. learning to become at home in the poet's proper domain   *Reviewing*
6. abiding or dwelling in the nearness of the homeland, near the primal source, near the origin   *Part[y]ing, Dying*

The journey is the dance, the place ballet, the interplay between movement and rest, between dwelling and mobility. There are moments of homecoming as returns enhanced, those aesthetic experiences when there is a feeling of a serenity of mood, a vividness of presence and a heightened self-awareness. And as the horizon of life draws near, there is peace in the heart of the home.

Returning enhanced to dwell on *The Dance to Death*

In this study, the return enhanced has been a feature of both the subject matter and the research process. By this I mean there were many instances and occasions during the actual research where I would discover an insight in the literature which was then put aside. Some months later I would return to the idea and the text with a renewed understanding of its relevance for the study. In writing, tensions occur when it is unclear where particular sections fit, and resolution when their rightful place is found. There was another tension at the start of the study about how German Idealism might appropriately be used here, but this has been resolved as I have come to understand the rhythmic patterns of the lifeworld through their "tension, intensity, and resolution" (Stephenson, 2005: 568). While this book is the product, Goethe would have recognised the reciprocal process of thinking and doing in its creation. For him "the link between reflection and experience, in which the aesthetic plays an essential mediating role, constituted the true basis of knowledge" (Bishop, 1999: 280). The tension of Jane's illness and death has been resolved for me in the process of reflecting on the experience.

This process of returning to previously considered but discarded scholarly texts, to then enhance understanding is similar to Gendlin's (2004) idea of experiencing as 'carrying forward'. That is when something is "the reaching behind itself in going forward … which is also the further implying that brings the further occurring" (Gendlin, 2004: 146). And this idea has been carried forward to suggest that "this kind of understanding is aesthetically inclusive and carries bodily felt implications" (Todres & Galvin, 2008: 573). So in feeling the tension between what I felt when caring for Jane, in remembering those times and in then using scholarly writing about that experience, I have perhaps achieved something akin to an 'aesthetic phenomenology in practice'. This is characterised by the principle "the aliveness of language and the empathic use of language to facilitate an experience of home-coming for others" (Todres & Galvin, 2008: 574). Earlier I stated that "I wanted the reader to have a strong sense of the visceral reality of advanced cancer", as the lifeworld is already "more than any category of already patterned knowing" (Todres & Galvin, 2008: 574). The challenge then is to find the language to describe this 'felt sense' of the experience which is "the direct referent, the implicit demanding" (Gendlin, 2004: 133). In turn this is reminiscent of Schiller's 'living form' which he describes in terms of a human being in *Letter 15*:

> As long as we merely think about his form, it is lifeless, a mere abstraction; as long as we merely feel his life, it is formless, a mere impression. Only when his form lives in our feeling and his life takes on form in our understanding, does he become living form; and this will always be the case when we adjudge him beautiful.[22]

Beauty in this sense is the aesthetic which in terms of Schiller's play-drive acts as a harmonising force between feelings and reason, where "through beauty we become truly human" (Bishop, 2008: 144). I hope therefore that in the aesthetic form of this book the reader will feel something of the 'living form' of Jane as she experienced her illness. In turn, the reader will reach an understanding of the role of the aesthetic for humanity.

The Dance to Death is now understood as the movement between the life necessitated by illness and 'normal' life, as it was otherwise known. The diagnosis of life-limiting illness can be interpreted as a turning point but, as I described earlier, it is more like a threshold and therefore an entrance to the sacred world of the dying. In this place it can be difficult for family and friends to know how to respond, therefore one of the contributions of this study is to demonstrate how the dance can work. The rich descriptions of daily life in *The Dance to Death* are contiguous with the Dwelling–Mobility lattice (Galvin & Todres, 2011a). This study has not attempted to validate the framework as such, but it has identified connections through the 'place ballet' of aesthetic experiences. The study has also hinted at the sense of homecoming that the bereaved partner might find through an active reappraisal of their shared experience of the life-limiting illness of a loved one. In the shared experience of life-limiting illness there is movement in the well-being of daily life and there is peacefulness, content to dwell at-home both spatially and experientially.

The final aspect of this study to highlight is the interpretation of aesthetic experience derived from the research. Aesthetic experience was defined as a feeling of serenity of mood, a vividness of presence and a heightened self-awareness. The case is made for particular aspects or characteristic dimensions which might enhance the appearance of such feelings. In the context of someone who is dying, these moments of exquisite wholeness may arise from sensations that are experienced in relation to particular places. Drawing on Simmel's notion of sociability and Turner's theory of communitas, these feelings may provide a sense of a return enhanced to everyday, secular life from the sacred place of dying. Awareness of the integrative nature of head, hand and heart avoids artificial contrivance and the spontaneity of aesthetic experience emerges naturally. The contributory aspects to the emergence of aesthetic experiences can be summarised as:

- a sense of at-homeness, a sacred, peaceful place – Heidegger, Seamon
- the inner court of family and friends that provides a context for sociability – Turner, Simmel
- heightened sensory awareness experienced as moments of pleasure through taste, touch, smell, sound and sight – Schiller, Simmel

This study has explored in some detail one woman's experience of ovarian cancer, from diagnosis to death. It has traced a path through that experience using insights drawn from eighteenth-century German literature as an understanding of the aesthetic. It is not a study of life and death but of living and dying with a spirit of well-being. This is encapsulated in the emergence of aesthetic experience through the related aspects of place, people and perception. Recalling the earlier reference to Goethe's world of beautiful imperfections is also a reminder of human finitude. In the context of Japanese culture and aesthetics, this is exemplified by the annual celebration of the cherry blossom as a symbol of life's impermanence (Juniper, 2003). As a study of life, love and loss, this book may well be full of beautiful imperfections. Better then to give Jane the last words "I admire the courage it takes to commit to paper how you feel about someone, what they have meant to you, what you have learned from them" (Blog post, 'So Much Love', day 330).

Notes

1 See Internet Movie Database entry for details: www.imdb.com/title/tt0825232/
2 See Chapter 3.
3 This observation has also been made by Strawson (2004: 441).
4 See Chapter 2: Finding.
5 See Chapter 4.
6 Marion Coutts: 'There is going to be a destruction … the obliteration of a person', *The Observer*, Sunday 15 June 2014. Available at: www.theguardian.com/books/2014/jun/15/marion-coutts-tom-lubbock-iceberg-extract
7 Tom Lubbock: 'A memoir of living with a brain tumour', *The Observer*, Sunday 7 November 2010. Available at: www.theguardian.com/books/2010/nov/07/tom-lubbock-brain-tumour-language
8 As an American author Carper uses this spelling throughout but I will use the more widely accepted 'aesthetics'.
9 Here my thinking is in a sense similar to Gendlin's (2004) idea of coming into words.
10 See the definition given in the first chapter from Schiller's *Letter 18* (WW: 123) where beauty provides the link between feeling and thinking.
11 WW: 310.
12 See Chapter 2: Wondering.
13 See Chapter 1: Aesthetic Letters. Yet I only realised this point when I revisited the thesis in preparation for this book.
14 WW: lxxxv.
15 See also the translator's preface of *Being and Time* (Heidegger, 1996).
16 See Chapter 1.
17 Stephenson, 2005.
18 First given as a lecture in 1954.
19 In one of his last works, Heidegger (1973) makes direct reference to Goethe's primal phenomenon in relation to space as an irreducible concept.
20 See Chapter 1: Schiller's aesthetic education.
21 See Chapter 2: Wondering.
22 WW: 101.

References

Allen, Davina & Lyne, Patricia (2006) *The Reality of Nursing Research: Politics, Practices and Processes*, London: Routledge

Arnold, Peter J (2005) 'Somaesthetics, education, and the art of dance', *The Journal of Aesthetic Education*, 39, 1, 48–64

Battani, Marshall (2011) 'Aura, self, and aesthetic experience', *Contemporary Aesthetics*, 9
Bishop, Paul (1999) 'Epistemological problems and aesthetic solutions in Goethe and Jung', *Goethe Yearbook*, 9, 278–317
Bishop, Paul (2008) *Analytical Psychology and German Classical Aesthetics: Goethe, Schiller, and Jung*, Volume 1: *The Development of the Personality*, London: Routledge
Bouchal, S R (2007) 'Moral meanings of caring for the dying', in N E Johnston & A Scholler-Jaquish, Eds, *Meaning in Suffering: Caring Practices in the Health Professions*, Madison: University of Wisconsin Press, 232–275
Bragg, Melvyn (2007) 'We tend to forget that life can only be defined in the present tense', *The Guardian*, 12 September
Brook, I (1998) 'Goethean science as a way to read landscape', *Landscape Research*, 23, 1, 51–69
Brook, I (2013) 'Aesthetic appreciation of landscape', in P Howard, I Thompson & E Waterton, Eds, *The Routledge Companion to Landscape Studies*, London: Routledge, 108–118
Bury, Mike (2001) 'Illness narratives: fact or fiction?', *Sociology of Health & Illness*, 23, 3, 263–285
Butler, Sandra & Rosenblum, Barbara (1991) *Cancer in Two Voices*, San Francisco: Spinsters Ink Books
Buttimer, Anne (1976) 'Grasping the dynamism of lifeworld', *Annals of the Association of American Geographers*, 66, 2, 277–292
Cameron, John (2005) 'Place, Goethe and Phenomenology: a theoretic journey', *Janus Head*, 8, 1, 174–198
Campbell, Joseph (1949/2012) *The Hero with a Thousand Faces*, San Francisco: New World Library
Carel, Havi (2011) 'Phenomenology and its application in medicine', *Theoretical Medicine & Bioethics*, 32, 1, 33–46
Carper, Barbara A (1978) 'Fundamental patterns of knowing in nursing', *Advances in Nursing Science*, 1, 13–24
Carroll, Noël (2002) 'Aesthetic experience revisited', *Journal of Aesthetic Education*, 42, 2, 145–168
Chinn, Peggy (1994) 'Developing a method for aesthetic knowing in nursing', in Peggy Chinn & Jean Watson, Eds, *Art & Aesthetics in Nursing*, New York: National League for Nurses
Chinn, Peggy L & Kramer, Maeona K (2010) *Integrated Theory & Knowledge Development in Nursing*, St Loius: Mosby, 8th edition
Clements, Paul T & Averill, Jennifer B (2006) 'Finding patterns of knowing in the work of Florence Nightingale', *Nursing Outlook*, 54, 5, 268–274
Copp, Gina (1996) *Facing Impending Death: The Experiences of Patients and their Nurses in a Hospice Setting*, PhD, Oxford: Oxford Brookes University
Copp, Gina (1998) 'A review of current theories of death and dying', *Journal of Advanced Nursing*, 28, 2, 382–390
Cotterell, Phil (2006) *Living with Life Limiting Conditions: A Participatory Study of People's Experiences and Needs*, PhD, Uxbridge: Brunel University
Cotterell, Phil, Findlay, Helen & Macfarlane, Ann (2009) 'Patient and carer narratives and stories', in Yasmin Gunaratnam & David Oliviere, Eds, *Narrative and Stories in Health Care*, Oxford: Oxford University Press, 127–139
Coutts, Marion (2014) *The Iceberg: A Memoir*, London: Atlantic Books
Davies, Bronwyn & Gannon, Susanne (2012) 'Collective biography and the entangled enlivening of being', *International Review of Qualitative Research*, 5, 4, 357–376
Davies, Michelle L (1997) 'Shattered assumptions: time and the experience of long-term HIV positivity', *Social Science & Medicine*, 44, 5, 561–571
Davis, Courtney (2015) 'Drugs, cancer and end-of-life care: a case study of pharmaceuticalization?', *Social Science & Medicine*, 131, 207–214

Derbyshire, Philip (1999) 'Nursing, art and science: revisiting the two cultures', *International Journal of Nursing Practice*, 5, 123–131

Dowling, Maura (2007) 'From Husserl to van Manen: a review of different phenomenological approaches', *International Journal of Nursing Studies*, 44, 131–142

Dreyfus, H L & Wrathall, M A (2004) 'Martin Heidegger: an introduction to his thought, work, and life', in H L Dreyfus & M A Wrathall, Eds, *A Companion to Heidegger*, Oxford: Blackwell Publishing

Eva, Gail & Paley, John (2006) 'Stories in palliative care', *Progress in Palliative Care*, 14, 4, 155–164

Field, David & Copp, Gina (1999) 'Communication and awareness about dying in the 1990s', *Palliative Medicine*, 13, 6, 459–468

Fisher, Pamela & Freshwater, Dawn (2014) 'Towards compassionate care through aesthetic rationality', *Scandinavian Journal Caring Science*, 28, 4, 767–774

Frank, Arthur W (2001) 'Can we research suffering?', *Qualitative Health Research*, 11, 353–362

Frank, Arthur W (2010) *Letting Stories Breathe: A Socio-narratology*, Chicago: University of Chicago Press

Frank, Arthur W (2013) *The Wounded Storyteller: Body, Illness, and Ethics*, Chicago: University of Chicago Press, 2nd edition

Frankl, V E (2004) *Man's Search for Meaning*, London: Rider

Fuente, Eduardo de la (2008) 'The art of social forms and the social forms of art: the sociology aesthetics nexus in Georg Simmel's thought', *Sociological Theory*, 26, 4, 344–362

Galvin, Kathleen & Todres, Les (2007) 'The creativity of "unspecialization": a contemplative direction for integrative scholarly practice', *Phenomenology & Practice*, 1, 31–46

Galvin, Kathleen & Todres, Les (2011a) 'Kinds of well-being: a conceptual framework that provides direction for caring', *International Journal of Qualitative Studies in Health & Well-being*, 6

Galvin, Kathleen & Todres, Les (2011b) 'Research based empathic knowledge for nursing: a translational strategy for disseminating phenomenological research findings to provide evidence for caring practice', *International Journal of Nursing Studies*, 48, 4, 522–530

Gaydos, H Lea Barbato (2006) 'The art of nursing', *Explore: The Journal of Science & Healing*, 2, 1, 70–74

Gendlin, E T (2004) 'The new phenomenology of carrying forward', *Continental Philosophy Review*, 37, 1, 127–151

Gerhardt, Uta (1991) 'Research note. The roles of the wife and marital reality construction in the narrative interview: conceptual models in qualitative data interpretation', *Sociology of Health & Illness*, 13, 3, 411–428

Gesler, Wilbert M (1992) 'Therapeutic landscapes: medical issues in light of the new cultural geography', *Social Science & Medicine*, 34, 7, 735–746

Gibbon, Lewis Grassic (2006) *A Scots Quair*, Edinburgh: Polygon

Gould, Philip (2012) *When I Die: Lessons from the Death Zone*, London: Little, Brown

Gubar, Susan (2012) *Memoir of a Debulked Woman: Enduring Ovarian Cancer*, New York: W W Norton & Co

Hammermeister, Kai (2000) 'Heimat in Heidegger and Gadamer', *Philosophy & Literature*, 24, 312–326

Haraway, D J (2003) *The Companion Species Manifesto: Dogs, People and Significant Otherness*, Chicago: Prickly Paradigm Press

Hawkins, Anne H (1993) *Reconstructing Illness: Studies in Pathography*, West Lafayette: Purdue University Press

Hawkins, Anne H (1999) 'Pathography: patient narratives of illness', *Western Journal of Medicine*, 171, 127–129

Heidegger, Martin (1973) 'Art and space', *Man & World*, 6, 3–8
Heidegger, Martin (1977) *Question Concerning Technology and Other Essays*, New York: Garland Publishing Inc.
Heidegger, Martin (1977) 'Science and reflection', in *Question Concerning Technology and Other Essays*, New York: Garland Publishing Inc., 155–182
Heidegger, Martin (1993) *Basic Writings: Martin Heidegger*, London: Routledge
Heidegger, Martin (1996) *Being and Time*, New York: State University of New York
Heidegger, Martin (2000) *Elucidations in Hölderlin's Poetry*, New York: Prometheus Books
Hydén, Lars-Christer (1997) 'Illness and narrative', *Sociology of Health & Illness*, 19, 1, 48–69
Jagodzinski, J & Wallin, J (2013) *Arts-based Research: A Critique and a Proposal*, Rotterdam: Sense Publishers
Jayde, V, Boughton, M & Blomfield, P (2013) 'The experience of chemotherapy-induced alopecia for Australian women with ovarian cancer', *European Journal of Cancer Care*, 22, 503–512
Jones, Howard (2014) 'The varieties of aesthetic experience', *Journal for Spiritual & Consciousness Studies*, 30, 114, 238–248
Joy, Annamma & Sherry, Jr, John F (2003) 'Speaking of art as embodied imagination: a multisensory approach to understanding aesthetic experience', *Journal of Consumer Research*, 30, 2, 259–282
Juniper, A (2003) *Wabi Sabi: The Japanese Art of Impermanence*, New York: Tuttle Publishing
Lakoff, George (1973) 'Hedges: a study in meaning criteria and the logic of fuzzy concepts', *Journal of Philosophical Logic*, 2, 4, 458–508
Law, John (2000) 'On the subject of the object: narrative, technology, and interpellation', *Configurations*, 8, 1, 1–29
Lee, Monica & Silver, Daniel (2013) 'Simmel's law of the individual and the ethics of the relational self', *Theory, Culture & Society*, 29, 7–8, 124–145
Leight, Susan B (2001) 'Starry night: using story to inform aesthetic knowing in women's health nursing', *Journal of Advanced Nursing*, 37, 1, 108–114
Lorde, Audre (1980) *The Cancer Journals*, San Fransisco: Aunt Lute Books
Lubbock, Tom (2012) *Until Further Notice, I Am Alive*, London: Granta Books
Maltoni, M & Amadori, D (2001) 'Palliative medicine and medical oncology', *Annals of Oncology*, 12, 4, 443–450
Mattingly, Cheryl (1998a) 'In search of the good: narrative reasoning in clinical practice', *Medical Anthropology Quarterly*, 12, 273–297
Mattingly, Cheryl (1998b) *Healing Dramas and Clinical Plots: The Narrative Structure of Experience*, Cambridge: Cambridge University Press
Mishler, Elliot G (1995) 'Models of narrative analysis: a typology', *Journal of Narrative & Life History*, 5, 2, 87–123
Morris, Sara M (2001) 'Joint and individual interviewing in the context of cancer', *Qualitative Health Research*, 11, 4, 553–567
Mugerauer, Robert (2008) *Heidegger and Homecoming: The Leitmotif in the Later Writings*, Toronto: University of Toronto Press
Murray, Scott A, Kendall, Marilyn, Boyd, Kirsty & Sheikh, Aziz (2005) 'Illness trajectories and palliative care', *British Medical Journal*, 330, 1007–1011
Neville, Michael R (1974) 'Kant's characterisation of aesthetic experience', *The Journal of Aesthetics & Art Criticism*, 33, 2, 193–202
Newbury, Margaret J (2009) *The Carer's Initiation: A Qualitative Study of the Experience of Family Care of the Dying*, Professional Doctorate in Health thesis, Bath: University of Bath
Payne, S, Brearley, S, Milligan, C, Seamark, D, Thomas, C, WangXu, Blake, S & Turner, M (2012) 'The perspectives of bereaved family carers on dying at home: the study

protocol of "unpacking the home" – family carers' reflections on dying at home', *BMC Palliative Care*, 11, 23

Pezze, Barbara Dalle (2006) 'Heidegger on Gelassenheit', *Minerva – An Internet Journal of Philosophy*, 10, 94–122; www.minerva.mic.ul.ie/vol10/Heidegger.pdf

Plenderleith, Helen Jane (1993) 'An approach to Goethe's treatment of religion in *Dichtung und Wahrheit*', *German Life & Letters*, 46, 297–310

Polak, Louisa & Green, Judith (2015) 'Using joint interviews to add analytic value', *Qualitative Health Research*, 26, 12, 1638–1648

Pugh, W T Gordon (1944) *Practical Nursing: Including Hygiene and Dietetics*, London: Blackwood

Pugh, W T Gordon (1969) *Practical Nursing*, London: Blackwood

Radcliffe, Eloise, Lowton, Karen & Morgan, Myfanwy (2013) 'Co-construction of chronic illness narratives by older stroke survivors and their spouses', *Sociology of Health & Illness*, 35, 7, 993–1007

Relph, Edward (1976) *Place and Placelessness*, London: Pion Ltd

Riessman, C K (2015) 'Ruptures and sutures: time, audience and identity in an illness narrative', *Sociology of Health & Illness*, 37, 7, 1055–1071

Riessman, C K & Speedy, J (2007) 'Narrative inquiry in the psychotherapy professions: a critical review' in D J Clandinin, Ed., *Handbook of Narrative Inquiry: Mapping a Methodology*, Thousand Oaks: SAGE Publications, 426–457

Robinson, Ian (1990) 'Personal narratives, social careers and medical courses: analysing life trajectories in autobiographies of people with multiple sclerosis', *Social Science & Medicine*, 30, 11, 1173–1186

Robinson, Mairi (1985) *The Concise Scots Dictionary*, Aberdeen: Aberdeen University Press

Rose, Gillian (1995) *Love's Work*, London: Chatto & Windus

Sakellariou, Dikaios, Boniface, Gail & Brown, Paul (2013) 'Using joint interviews in a narrative-based study on illness experiences', *Qualitative Health Research*, 23, 11, 1563–1570

Schindler, D C (2008) 'An aesthetics of freedom: Friedrich Schiller's breakthrough beyond subjectivism', *Yearbook of the Irish Philosophical Society*, 84–109

Seamon, David (1979) *A Geography of the Lifeworld: Movement, Rest, and Encounter*, London: Croom Helm

Seamon, David (1998) 'Goethe, nature and phenomenology', in David Seamon, & Arthur Zajonc, Eds, *Goethe's Way of Science: A Phenomenology of Nature*, Albany, NY: State University of New York Press

Seamon, David (2005) 'Goethe's way of science as a phenomenology of nature', *Janus Head*, 8, 1, 86–101

Sharpe, Lesley (1991) *Friedrich Schiller: Drama, Thought and Politics*, Cambridge: Cambridge University Press

Sheehan, T (2004) 'Dasein', in H L Dreyfus & M A Wrathall, Eds, *A Companion to Heidegger*, Oxford: Blackwell Publishing Ltd

Shusterman, Richard (1997) 'The end of aesthetic experience', *The Journal of Aesthetics & Art Criticism*, 55, 29–41

Shusterman, Richard (1999) 'Somaesthetics: a disciplinary proposal', *Journal of Aesthetics & Art Criticism*, 299–313

Shusterman, Richard (2006) 'Aesthetic experience: from analysis to Eros', *The Journal of Aesthetics & Art Criticism*, 64, 2, 217–229

Shusterman, Richard (2011) 'Soma, self, and society: somaesthetics as pragmatist meliorism', *Metaphilosophy*, 42, 3, 314–327

Shusterman, Richard & Tomlin, Adele (2010) *Aesthetic Experience*, London: Routledge

Siles-Gonzalez, Jose & Solano-Ruiz, Carmen (2015) 'Sublimity and beauty: a view from nursing aesthetics', *Nursing Ethics*, 1–13

Simmel, Georg & Hughes, Everett C (1949) 'The sociology of sociability', *American Journal of Sociology*, 55, 3, 254–261

Simmel, Georg (1997) 'The sociology of the meal', in D Frisby & M Featherstone, Eds, *Simmel on Culture: Selected Writings*, London: SAGE Publications, 130–135

Simms, Eva-Maria (2005) 'Goethe, Husserl, and the crisis of the European Sciences', *Janus Head*, 8, 1, 160–172

SOED (2007) *Shorter Oxford English Dictionary*, Oxford: Oxford University Press

Sontag, S (1978) *Illness as Metaphor*, Harmondsworth: Penguin

Stephenson, Roger H (2005) '"Binary synthesis": Goethe's aesthetic intuition in literature and science', *Science in Context*, 18, 4, 553–581

Stewart, Isla & Cuff, Herbert E (1899) *Practical Nursing*, Edinburgh: William Blackwood

Strawson, Galen (2004) 'Against narrativity', *Ratio*, 17, 4, 428–452

Svenaeus, Fredrik (2003) 'Das Unheimliche: towards a phenomenology of illness', *Medicine, Health Care, & Philosophy*, 3, 3–16

Thompson, Kimberly (2007) 'Liminality as a descriptor for the cancer experience', *Illness, Crisis & Loss*, 15, 333–351

Timmermans, Stefan (1994) 'Dying of awareness: the theory of awareness contexts revisited', *Sociology of Health & Illness*, 16, 322–339

Todres, Les & Galvin, Kathleen (2008) 'Embodied interpretation: a novel way of evocatively re-presenting meanings in phenomenological research', *Qualitative Research*, 8, 5, 568–583

Todres, Les & Galvin, Kathleen (2010) '"Dwelling-mobility": an existential theory of well-being', *International Journal of Qualitative Studies in Health & Well-being*, 5, 3

Tomlin, A (2010) 'Introduction', in R Shusterman & A Tomlin, Eds, *Aesthetic Experience*, London: Routledge

Turner, Edith (2012) *Communitas: The Anthropology of Collective Joy*, London: Palgrave Macmillan

Turner, Victor (1969) *The Ritual Process*, Ithaca: Cornell University Press

van Gennep, Arnold (1960) *The Rites of Passage*, London: Routledge & Kegan Paul

Wainwright, Paul (2000) 'Towards an aesthetics of nursing', *Journal of Advanced Nursing*, 32, 3, 750–756

Wilkinson, E M & Willoughby, L A (1967) *On the Aesthetic Education of Man in a Series of Letters*, Oxford: Clarendon Press

Williams, Simon J, Martin, Paul & Gabe, Jonathan (2011) 'The pharmaceuticalisation of society? A framework for analysis', *Sociology of Health & Illness*, 33, 5, 710–725

Wojnar, Danuta M & Swanson, Kristen M (2007) 'Phenomenology: an exploration', *Journal of Holistic Nursing*, 25, 3, 172–180

Woods, Angela (2011) 'The limits of narrative: provocations for the medical humanities', *Medical Humanities*, 37, 2, 73–78

Woods, A (2012) 'Beyond the wounded storyteller: rethinking narrativity, illness and embodied self-experience' in H Carel & R Cooper, Eds, *Health, Illness and Disease*, Durham: Acumen Publishing

Zander, Patricia E (2007) 'Ways of knowing in nursing: the historical evolution of a concept', *The Journal of Theory Construction & Testing*, 11, 1, 7–11

INDEX

Adamson, Veronica x, 2, 5, 35
aesthetic discourse 19–21, 177
aesthetic experience 15–16, 167–70, 173–6, 179–80, 182; definition 173
aesthetic intuition 24–5
aesthetic phenomenology 25, 27, 34, 181
alopecia *see* hair loss
art of nursing 26, 165
ascites 55, 131–2
at-homeness 151, 172–3, 176, 182
autobiography 2–4, 26, 28, 29, 152
autoethnography 2, 31, 97

battle 26, 101
Beiser, Frederick 7–8, 10, 12, 15
Bentley, Susan 15, 17
bereavement 2, 182, 186
Bildungsroman 25, 28–9, 153
binary synthesis x, 4, 21–3
Bishop, Paul 18, 26, 169, 181–82
Bochner, Arthur 2, 31
Bortoft, Henri 17–19
boundaries 27–8
bricolage x–xi
Brook, Isis 179
bucket list 148–9
buffering 102, 106
burden 78–9, 89, 109
Bury, Michael 79, 105, 154
Butler, Sandra 65, 160–2

Campbell, Joseph 153, 156
Carel, Havi 72, 168

carer performance 100–1, 104–5
Carper, Barbara A 164–6, 183
Charon, Rita xi, 2, 7
chemo bunnet 85, 157
Clandinin, D Jean 30–1
communitas 140, 173, 175, 182
companion stories 1, 148–9, 151, 164
confidentiality x, 26, 32, 119, 174
Copp, Gina 104, 132, 143, 161–2
Coutts, Marion 65, 160, 162–4, 175–6
Craig, Charlotte 9–10

Dance to Death 43, 48, 76, 111, 116, 182; Wondering 48, 180, 183; Finding 57, 183; Planning 65, 180; Treating 76, 152, 180; Turning 90, 144, 180; Living 100, 180; Reviewing 116, 144, 155, 180; Part[y]ing 126, 180; Dying 136, 180
dance metaphor 5–6, 64, 79, 87, 104, 110, 170
denial 50, 58, 62, 95–6, 158
dialectic 53, 61, 72, 79
Dickinson, Emily 109–10
documents of life xi, 32–5
dwelling 172–3, 176–80

Ellis, Carolyn 2, 31
embodied relational understanding 27, 43, 144
enhancement 13, 22, 159, 167
epistemology 28–9, 36

Fichte, Johann Gottlieb 9–10, 14
fiction 25–6

field text 30, 32–3
Frank, Arthur 1, 29, 117, 142, 145, 147–9, 151–8, 161, 166
French Revolution 9, 11
Froggatt, Katherine 6, 27, 127, 130, 140–1
Furber, Lynn 109–10, 121

Gadamer, Hans-Georg x, 12, 49, 80, 172
Galvin, Kate 24–25, 27, 31, 34, 43, 148, 151, 170, 176, 180–2
Gegnet 178, 180
Gendlin, Eugene 24–5, 27, 181, 183
German: language 4, 7, 22, 35; literature xi, 28, 47, 182; Idealism 7–9; Romanticism 9, 26
Gestalt 19–20, 169
Goethe, Johann Wolfgang: *Anschauung* 20, 23–4; aesthetics 20–4, 170–1; *Dichtung und Wahrheit* 4; *Faust* 11, 26, 80; maxims 4, 21; relationship with Schiller 10–11, 20–1, 169–70, 177; science 17–19, 26, 171; Polarity 23; Theory of Colour 18–19, 177; *Urpflanze* 18; *Urphenomenon* 8, 18–21, 177–8
Goldbeck, Rainer 58, 95
Grassic Gibbon, Lewis 179–80
guarding 55, 83, 102–3
Gubar, Susan 147, 153

hair loss 7, 67, 79, 83–7, 157
Hammermeister, Kai 9, 12–14, 178
Hawkins, Anne 26, 153
health records 32–3, 72–3, 119–20, 144
Heidegger, Martin 24, 28, 34, 53, 168, 173, 176–80, 182–3
Heimat 53, 178, 180
Hölderlin 177–8, 180
home 46, 53–4, 60, 130, 159, 171–3, 175–80
hope 97–98
horizon 49, 172
hospice care 27, 96, 130, 140–1, 161, 163, 175–6
humanistic geography 171–2

illness narrative 25, 29, 143, 148, 154–60, 187
Illness Period xii, 5, 32, 43, 51, 116, 144
illness writing 7, 25–6, 148
interviews: purpose of 31–4; self-directed 24, 32
interviewer 31–4
irony 7, 60–1

Jena, University of 8, 10, 17
Jung, Carl G 81, 142

Kant, Immanuel 9–10; *Critique of Judgement* 9, 12
Kellehear, Allan 8, 96
Kubler-Ross, Elizabeth 96

Lakoff, George 6, 178
Lambek, Michael 7, 60–1
landscape 16, 26, 179
Langellier, Kristin M, 27, 31
lifeworld 172, 179, 181
liminal 27, 53, 60, 130, 142, 175
Long, Judy 109
Lubbock, Tom 160, 163

Mann, Thomas 25–6, 101
Mattingly, Cheryl 78, 148, 160
metaphor 5–7, 155–7
Morse, Janice 83, 101–2, 106
Mugerauer, Robert 176–8, 180

narrative inquiry 24–5, 29–32
narrative types 154; automythological 153, 155, 157; chaos 151, 153–6, 158, 161; manifesto 153, 155–6; memoir 153, 155, 161, 170, 175; quest 151, 153, 155–8; restitution 151, 153–5, 158, 161
Newbury, Margaret J 65, 100–1, 160
nursing practice 1, 164, 167

ontology 28–9, 36, 176, 178
open awareness 97–8, 161, 163
optimism 3, 98, 118
ovarian cancer 49, 68–71, 84, 92, 94, 107, 153

palliative care 27, 98, 160, 162
pathography 26, 153
Payne, Sheila 27, 110, 125, 160
peritoneal drain 127, 131, 133
phenomenology x, 12, 24–5, 27, 170–2, 177, 181
place ballet 172, 180, 182
Plenderleith, Jane ix, xi, 3–4, 8–9, 20–2, 61, 171
Plummer, Ken xi–xii, 34
poetry 20–1, 177–8, 180
polarity 5, 15, 22–3, 80–1, 171
presence 169, 173
PTSD 92–3

Reed, TJ 10–11, 18
reinvention 85, 153, 155, 157
return enhanced ix, 4, 21–3
Riessman, Catherine K 24, 29–30, 155
Rosenblum, Barbara 59, 65, 160–2
ruling relations 106, 117

Schaper, Eva 12–14
Schiller, Friedrich: *Aesthetic Letters* 4, 13–16, 21–2, 35–6, 169; aesthetics 9–12, 169–71; basic drives 14–15, 174; beauty 9–13, 15–16, 35, 182–3; *Die Horen* 10, 13; *Kallias Letters* 12, 35, 169; living form 11, 28, 181–2; relationship with Goethe 10–11, 20–1, 169–70, 177; third thing 14, 23
Schindler, DC 12, 169, 171, 178
Schmitz, L Dora 11, 16
Scotland 44, 46–9
Seamon, David 19, 171–73, 179, 182
self-esteem 62, 95, 135
Sharpe, Lesley 9–10, 12, 16–18, 35, 170
Shotter, John 28
Shusterman, Richard 168–9
Simmel, Georg 174–5, 182
Smith, Dorothy E 106, 117
Snyder, CR 98
sociability 173–5, 182
somaesthetics 168
Sontag, Susan 6, 155
Speedy, Jane 29–30, 155
Stacey, Jackie 6, 64, 93
Stanley, Liz xi, 4, 12, 28–30

Stephenson, Roger 17–23, 36n24, 170–1, 177, 180–1
storyboard 33–4
Svenaeus, Fredrik 53, 54, 171
symbolism 80–1, 150, 183

Taoism 5
terror management theory 62
Timmermans, Stefan 97–8, 161
Todres, Les 24–5, 27, 31, 34, 43, 148, 151, 170, 176, 180–2
tuberculosis 25, 101, 159
Turner, Victor 142, 175, 182

van Manen, Max x, 24, 28,
Voltaire 3

Wagner, Richard 80–1; *Parsifal* 79–81, 118, 142
Weimar Classicism 9
Wengraf, Tom 31–32
Wilkinson, Elizabeth M 11–14, 16–17, 20–2, 35n2, 36n28, 173
Willoughby, Leonard 11–14, 16–17, 20–2, 35n2, 36n28, 173
Wilson, Sharon 83, 101–2, 106
Woods, Angela 151, 158
Woolf, Virginia 26

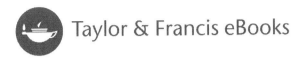# Taylor & Francis eBooks

Helping you to choose the right eBooks for your Library

Add Routledge titles to your library's digital collection today. Taylor and Francis ebooks contains over 50,000 titles in the Humanities, Social Sciences, Behavioural Sciences, Built Environment and Law.

Choose from a range of subject packages or create your own!

Benefits for you
- Free MARC records
- COUNTER-compliant usage statistics
- Flexible purchase and pricing options
- All titles DRM-free.

Benefits for your user
- Off-site, anytime access via Athens or referring URL
- Print or copy pages or chapters
- Full content search
- Bookmark, highlight and annotate text
- Access to thousands of pages of quality research at the click of a button.

 Free Trials Available
We offer free trials to qualifying academic, corporate and government customers.

eCollections – Choose from over 30 subject eCollections, including:

Archaeology	Language Learning
Architecture	Law
Asian Studies	Literature
Business & Management	Media & Communication
Classical Studies	Middle East Studies
Construction	Music
Creative & Media Arts	Philosophy
Criminology & Criminal Justice	Planning
Economics	Politics
Education	Psychology & Mental Health
Energy	Religion
Engineering	Security
English Language & Linguistics	Social Work
Environment & Sustainability	Sociology
Geography	Sport
Health Studies	Theatre & Performance
History	Tourism, Hospitality & Events

For more information, pricing enquiries or to order a free trial, please contact your local sales team:
www.tandfebooks.com/page/sales

 The home of Routledge books

www.tandfebooks.com